Children with Language Disorders

This book is dedicated to
Matthew and Katie, who have already said so much,
and Jennifer, who is just getting started.

Children with Language Disorders

Janet Lees, MSc, LCST

Consultant Speech Therapist
Newcomen Centre, Guy's Hospital, London

Shelagh Urwin, MPhil, LCST

Lecturer and Community Speech Therapist
City University, London

Whurr Publishers
London and New Jersey

Copyright © Janet Lees and Shelagh Urwin 1991
First published by
Whurr Publishers Limited
19b Compton Terrace
London N1 2UN
England

First published 1991

Reprinted 1991

British Library Cataloguing in Publication Data

Lees, Janet
  Children with language disorders.
  1. Children. Speech disorders. Therapy
  I. Title   II. Urwin, Shelagh
  618.9285506

  ISBN 1-870332-61-X

Phototypeset by Scribe Design, Gillingham, Kent
Printed in Great Britain by Athenaeum Press, Newcastle upon Tyne

Introduction

Each year a number of new texts appear on the subject of language-impaired children. Any reader of this one might reasonably ask in what way it differs from others. Principally, this text aims to approach the subject from the clinical perspective. It is written by two speech therapists and it aims to set out what speech therapists, working individually and in multidisciplinary teams, really do with language-impaired children. In pursuit of that aim it discusses real language-impaired children, their difficulties and needs. Working from the clinical perspective, various theoretical models of language and recent research findings are then discussed. By this method the book aims to illustrate an holistic view of the child, her or his family, environment and progress with language.

This approach draws upon clinical questions which we have posed, or which have been put to us by students, various professionals and parents concerned with language-impaired children. It has been developed in a range of clinical settings including child development centres, language units and community clinics. It has been tested in research studies and discussed by colleagues and students of many disciplines and reflected on in the course of further work and observation. In all of these respects the work is ongoing and has not ceased with the publication of this book. We are concerned to demonstrate the value of an holistic clinical approach which includes the objective and logical alongside the subjective and intuitive. In our view this is how speech therapists work in clinical practice. There is considerable value in this approach if it is discussed and evaluated.

Essentially this book is about making connections. We have set out to make connections between clinical practice, theoretical models and research. In making these connections we have aimed to keep the language-impaired child central to our discussion and understanding. Keeping the child's needs central to practice leads on to three fundamental connections: working with success, working with the family and working with others. Whenever we discuss clinical methods of assessment, diagnosis or treatment for language-impaired children, we urge that this should be done so that the child has an ongoing experience of success. Too many of our children live and work with failure as a common experience. If we are to be active in the process by which language-impaired children may develop their full potential, success will be an important factor in generating motivation and raising self-esteem.

Language-disordered children do not exist in isolation. They live as a part of a 'family' unit in the broadest sense of the word. It is the people who make up this unit who are the first and most important people for the child to be able to communicate with. Therefore, despite the difficulties which it may entail, we urge an approach in which parents/carers and professionals work in partnership. Equally language-impaired children rarely present without additional needs which means that a wide range of professionals is usually involved in their care. Our third connection is therefore a need to work together. Whilst we recognise that not every working environment encourages a team approach to the management of language-impaired children, we wish to stress the benefits of team working. We would like to encourage clinicians to move away from a very individualistic approach to explore the challenge of working in a team. Only our openness to working with others will allow us all to develop a greater understanding of the needs of language-impaired children.

One of the advantages of working in a team is the way in which it becomes easier to help others to understand what therapy with language-impaired children is. We have continually found it difficult to explain, but it can be demonstrated. When discussing therapy that takes place in an open and creative environment, we are struck by the complexity of the therapeutic relationship. When asked what the fundamental requirements for good therapy with language-impaired children are, the first answer is a flexible imagination. Much has been said about the way in which therapy cannot be objectively described. It is a subjective experience which seems to rely heavily on intuition. Whilst not wishing to ignore our need to consider ways of being more objective and evaluating in our work, we also affirm the value of subjective thinking and intuition in the therapeutic process. However, it is not enough to leave it at that. We must consider what this means in practice. For us, it means that a fundamental part of the process of therapy with a language-impaired child is concerned with the therapist's ability to identify with the child's situation, enter into the child's experience and actively take part in learning with the child. By doing this the therapist will take the same steps as the child and actively live through the therapy programme step by step. In this way the question of speed and complexity of tasks is naturally encountered by both parties and set by common consent. The question of patience on the part of the therapist does not arise as she or he is intimately involved in the whole process and can feel the needs and frustrations of the child thus tuning the programme to the child's needs. It is not then necessary to respond with exasperation about the last 30 minutes spent achieving very little on a task. The therapist has long since recognised the need to modify it so that the child continues to learn creatively within the rewarding situation.

In the nine chapters of this book we have tried to expand this view of speech therapy with language-disordered children. In Chapter 1, we outline the concepts of delayed and deviant language development as we understand them, and discuss the development of a more appropriate terminology to describe the language problems we see in clinical practice. In particular we try to define language disorder by inclusion, rather than by exclusion as is usually the case. In other words we try to say what we think it is rather than what it is not. Chapter 2 details methods used by speech therapists and others to assess the language difficulties of children, both formally and informally. The tests mentioned are not intended to be a complete catalogue of those available but are selected from experience. Equally the informal methods of assessment which are described are ones which have worked for us.

The complex nature of language disorder and the way this affects the developing child is of concern to a wide range of professionals. In Chapter 3, we discuss how these professionals can work together in a multidisciplinary team for the effective differential diagnosis of the child's strengths and needs. The speech therapists' role in such a process is particularly emphasised. The following three chapters (4, 5 and 6) consider the management of language-disordered children in three age groups: the preschool child, the school-aged child and teenagers. Most of the strategies used will not be new or novel to many readers – we do not claim that they are. Rather, they are presented here as examples of therapeutic practice which have been useful to us. We hope that this will serve to encourage others to discuss what has been useful for them so that we might move forward in our understanding of the management of these children.

Indeed, it is this moving forward that forms the focus of Chapters 7 and 8. In Chapter 7 the discussion is about the things which can be brought into clinical practice to make it more efficient and more flexible to the needs of these children. Chapter 8 considers appropriate methods of clinically based research more formally. Finally, Chapter 9 is concerned with those children who present with acquired language problems. For those unfamiliar with this problem, it may seem a small group of little significance. However, both for those affected and in respect of our future understanding of language disorder, we cannot afford to judge this as a fringe issue. Following Chapter 9, there are two appendices: the first outlines a number of syndromes in which speech and language impairment are a part of the presenting problem; the second gives an example of a story-telling test that can be used to elicit a language sample.

Throughout the book the text includes descriptions of a total of 24 cases of children with language disorders. Whilst we do not claim that this represents the entire range of the problem, these cases seek to illustrate the points made by drawing on examples of actual clinical practice. Professionals working with language disorder will, we hope, recognise many similarities between the children represented here and those they meet in their own work. We recognise the difficulty of trying to represent the dynamic therapy situation in words and sentences. However, we hope that these descriptions will serve to alert others to the way children present and develop with language problems.

This text has been a number of years in the making and grew out of a friendship that is much valued by us both. One of the key points in its development was brought about by an opportunity to share in lecturing to speech therapy students at the City University, London. We would like to thank the members of the department there for their continuing support. Much of the clinical work discussed here was carried out at the John Horniman Preschool Language Unit, Worthing and the Newcomen Child Development Centre, at Guy's Hospital, London. It was within these multidisciplinary teams that the value of working together was discovered and firmly reinforced. We would also like to thank speech therapists from all parts of the South East Thames Region for referring children and discussing them with us. Much of what is written here has grown out of meetings, visits, shared assessments and discussions and we thank them for their enthusiasm. It is always difficult to thank individuals when so many have made important contributions. However, we would like to mention two people, as representative of all our colleagues, who have made working with language-disordered children such an exciting challenge. They are first Shirley Jackson, who worked so closely with Shelagh that many ideas about joint working in the classroom situation were developed and discussed between them. Secondly, Gillian Baird, who taught Janet so much about child development and with whom many fascinating children with language disorders have been seen. They are two of the many colleagues of different disciplines without whom our understanding of language disorder would be much the poorer.

An undertaking of this size would not have been possible in our hectic lives without a shared sense of fun and the support of others. Shelagh Urwin's husband, Gary, and Mum and Dad, are to be thanked for getting the Sunday dinner on the table on a number of occasions and for their full commitment to family life which made this possible. Janet Lees's family and support network are particularly thanked for the prayers that kept us going, especially through the times that made us wonder why we had started in the first place. We are particularly grateful to Shirley Jackson and Bob

Warwicker for their help with editing the text. Now we look forward to the next stage in our development, mindful of all that we have learned from language-disordered children.

Janet Lees, Oxford
Shelagh Urwin, Hurstpierpoint
1990

Contents

List of Cases

List of Abbreviations

ACA	acquired childhood aphasia
AVM	arteriovenous malformation
CELF	Clinical Evaluation of Language Function
CT	computed tomography
CVA	cerebrovascular accident
GCE	General Certificate of Education
GCS	Glasgow Coma Score
GCSE	General Certificate of Secondary Education
ITPA	Illinois Test of Psycholinguistic Ability
PICAC	Porch Index of Communicative Ability in Children
RDLS	Reynell Developmental Language Scales
TROG	Test for Reception of Grammar
TWF	Test of Word Finding
WFVT	Word Finding Vocabulary Test
WISC-R	Weschler Intelligence Scale for Children – Revised

Chapter 1
The Language-impaired Child

Summary

This chapter presents an outline of the concepts of delayed and deviant language development as they may be understood from a clinical perspective, a discussion of the development of a more appropriate terminology to describe the language problems seen in clinical practice, with an emphasis on the definition of language disorder by inclusion, rather than by exclusion.

Introduction

A quick look at the caseload of any speech therapist in general paediatric practice would reveal a wide range of children both in age and presenting problems. Most of them are likely to be under 5 years of age and therefore passing through a period recognised as important for all aspects of their development, including language. A description of any of these children would include the strengths and weaknesses of their communication development as a basis for decisions about any speech therapy intervention. On the surface, the child's problems could be related to difficulty in motor control, e.g. cerebral palsy, or a structural problem, like cleft palate, or sensory deficits, including visual or hearing problems, but this is not always the whole picture. Some of the children may seem to have more difficulties in one area of development than another, but it is more often the interaction of these which leads to the presenting clinical problem.

Difficulties in the development of language will be a recognised feature in the majority of these young children. If other children were to be described, a wider range of these strengths and weaknesses would be added. In deciding priorities for this caseload, the clinician will be comparing children: these numerous descriptions ultimately furnish us

1

with a broad spectrum of language skills and patterns of development. From this clinical description most speech therapists go on to select their priorities of management. It is precisely this incredible range and variation, both in the individual features of language and their rate of change, which has contributed to the clinical dilemma so well described by Coombes (1987):

> As always, questions facing clinicians fall into four categories:
> 1. How to know what to do
> 2. What to do (including who to do it to and where)
> 3. When to do it
> 4. When to stop. (p. 357)

It is the what, when, who, how and where of speech therapy with language-impaired children which will be discussed. In order to enter such a debate, it is necessary to decide what we mean by language impairment in childhood – how this notion has been and is developing. First two case histories of children who have received speech therapy will be considered.

Case 1

Referred at the age of 2 years by her GP, this child had incontinentia pigmenti (see Appendix I) with the result that she only had one, peg-like, deciduous tooth (an upper canine). She was under the care of a dentist who, together with the GP, sought an explanation for her delay in speech and language development. She uttered no clear words although her comprehension appeared good.

She was the second child of two healthy, unrelated parents. Her only sibling was an older brother, also healthy with no developmental problems. There was no family history of speech and language difficulty and no early developmental problems other than incontinentia pigmenti. Her hearing was normal and all other aspects of her development were well within the normal range. Her verbal comprehension was assessed using the Reynell Developmental Language Scales – Revised (Reynell, 1977) and was also within the normal range. During the assessment she made a few unintelligible sounds which did not appear to relate to specific items.

The therapist and mother discussed some ways of encouraging her expressive language development and a home programme was prepared. This was reviewed at monthly intervals for the first 3 months, when it became clear that her expressive language development was improving. She was then reviewed at 3-monthly intervals for 6 months and then 6-monthly intervals until she was 4 years old. During this time no further deciduous teeth appeared.

She was speaking in sentences and her sound system also developed normally except for a tendency to 'front' certain 'back' sounds (i.e. k and g were produced as t and d – this is a common process in the development of speech sound contrasts). At 4 years of age an upper denture was fitted which greatly increased her self-confidence and by the time she was seen again at 5 years of age there were no other speech and language difficulties.

Case 2

This 2-year-old child was referred by the developmental paediatrician at the local child development centre. There was a history of physical abuse within the family, and she and her older brother had both been taken into care. The older brother was also known to have a speech and language problem, and attended a language unit in another district. She was very withdrawn and appeared to have difficulty understanding what was said as well as having little speech. A hearing test revealed a moderate conductive loss and she had ventilation tubes (grommets) inserted for this. The rest of her development with the exception of play appeared to be within the normal range, although it was also difficult to hold her attention.

With the cooperation of her foster parents, a programme of therapy was started which concentrated on providing activities to improve play, attention, comprehension and expressive language within the framework of the Wolfson programme (described in Cooper, Moodley and Reynell, 1974). By the time she was 3 years old, and had been placed with adoptive parents, it was clear that she had a serious language problem. Although she had made some progress in all the areas mentioned, it was felt that there was still a marked mismatch between speech and language skills and other aspects of development which would mean that she would need special education by the time she was 5 years old. A statement of educational needs was prepared by the local educational psychologist in accordance with the 1981 Education Act. As a result of this she was placed in a preschool language unit at the age of 4 and remained there until she was 7 years old, when she was transferred to a further language unit placement. At that time her comprehension remained severely impaired and her expressive language was restricted to two- and three-word phrases which were unintelligible.

Both of the children described in Cases 1 and 2 are language impaired, but they are also very different. It is clear that whilst the first child had significant problems when referred at the age of 2 years, this was no longer a problem by the time she was 5 years old. The second child, however, had a problem that appears to be more extensive, both in the range of language skills affected and the severity. Progress was slower and there were still significant problems at the age of 7 years.

Children whose language development follows the same trend as the first case are usually described as having delayed language development. Children whose language development would align them with the second case might be described as having disordered or deviant language development. Not everyone concerned with language-impaired children accepts the delayed vs disordered notion in child language development. It is important to look at this debate because it affects our view of language-impaired children.

Normal vs Delayed Language Development

A discussion of the concept of delayed language development depends on the clear ideas of what normal language development is, what the acceptable range might be and how language development relates to other aspects of the child's development. There are a number of ways to describe the process of normal language development but two of the most common are using an age-related method and a skills-related model.

An age-related method

This suggests that a child should have mastered certain skills by a certain age. The major period for the development of language, say up to 5 years, is divided into age bands, and the progress which can be expected in each band is discussed. Usually the age bands fall closer together in the early stages and gradually become wider as the child gets older. Some variations to this method include a projected age range that tries to account for the variability within the population by suggesting what the upper and lower age limits of the acquisition of a particular level might be. The Stycar Sequences (Sheridan, 1973) use this basic method, proposing skills which can be observed in the normal child at 1, 3, 6, 9, 12, 15 and 18 months and then 2, 2½, 3, 4 and 5 years of age. Whilst this affords an easy comparison with the child's peers, it has disadvantages: it puts an emphasis on developmental delay and suggests that all that is required for the child to reach normal levels is an acceleration in development. Where a mismatch is found between certain skills, such that one age level is attributed to one skill and another age level to a different skill, it suggests that all that is required is greater input into the deficient area for the child to 'catch up'.

A *skills-related model*

With this model a child's development can be considered as the acquisition of certain skills that run parallel to each other and, to some extent, have an overlap or interdependency. Many well-known ways of describing language development choose this approach (Bloom and Lahey, 1978; Cooper, Moodley and Reynell, 1978; Bishop and Mogford, 1988), although the skills which each one discusses vary. Cooper, Moodley and Reynell (1978) consider the development of prelinguistic skills, symbolic understanding, verbal comprehension, expressive language and use of language for problem solving. Bloom and Lahey (1978) emphasise the development of language content, form and use, and the way in which these are related. Bishop and Mogford (1988) consider the various subsystems of language from a linguistic point of view. Thus, they describe the development of phonology (the development of speech–sound contrasts), syntax and morphology (grammatical development), semantics (the development of meaning) and pragmatics (the development of language use).

Each of these three models also considers the way in which the development of these separate and parallel skills interacts so that the child can achieve language competence. The disadvantage of a skills-related model is that it is possible to believe that, by concentrating on one particularly deficient skill, it is possible to accelerate progress in other areas of skill or that more general progress will be made through the interaction of these skills.

It is not our intention to detail yet another overview of language development; the reader is referred to the literature mentioned above for that. Indeed, the importance of considering a range of views on the development of language cannot be sufficiently emphasised. Language development is one area of study in which a narrow view which claims ascendancy over all others (some kind of 'therapeutic fundamentalism') is rarely helpful in the long term. The field is broad and children with language impairments all present as unique individuals. Therefore a wide vision is required of professionals working in this domain. A view of language development which emphasises the development of related and parallel skills within an age range-related framework that can be considered, alongside other areas of a child's development, to obtain a holistic picture of each language-impaired individual should be encouraged.

However, there are two major points which should be made about normal language development in relation to our understanding of language impairment in childhood. First is our growing understanding of the importance of the prelinguistic period for the child's future development.

There has been a growing body of research in this area, and it is clear that the infant has a wealth of communication skill well before the emergence of first words. It is also clear, when understanding deviant language development, that very early communication skills may be missing in some children. The following two questions about prelinguistic communication have been the subject of research:

1. How do infants make themselves understood?
2. What implications do prelinguistic skills have for language development?

Communication requires an initiator and a receiver; the parent/carer and the child alternate these roles. What begins as a series of innate signals develops through opportunities for interaction into an increasingly complex and elaborate repertoire of preverbal exchange. There are several elementary units of preverbal communicative activity, which include eye gaze, gesture and early vocalisation. These are initially used singly, but by the end of the first year they are coordinated into a range of sequences of reciprocal exchange with parents/carers. These sequences are rule governed, and the process by which the children understand the rules governing their composition and coordination is related to affective, social and cognitive development.

Affect

The infant appears to be born with a repertoire of affective behaviours which allow her or him to express basic needs. These innate behaviours ensure that the infant can elicit appropriate nuturing responses from the parent/carer. The infant initially responds to stimuli in the environment in terms of physical properties, such as size or brightness and, by 6 weeks, he or she begins to respond to the content of the events, e.g. as either pleasant or unpleasant. By 2 months, a smile will be the response to familiar people and objects. The child is now able to retrieve events and make comparisons, and also has the expectation that an event can be enjoyable.

The infant is not a passive partner but is actively involved in shaping exchanges with the parent/carer. While interacting both partners develop a recognition of the rules of these early exchanges. When appropriate events in the exchange are omitted or changed, the violation of the rule will lead to a change in the partner's behaviour.

Timing and turn-taking

An intrinsic part of this early communication, and one that is closely associated to affect, is a rhythmic compatibility that exists between infants and their parent/carer. The basic rhythms associated with primary needs develop a relation to environmental events as the infant becomes capable of directing actions towards an end (person or object). By about 2 months of age, interactions show the beginnings of regular reciprocal exchanges. Vocal and motor play develop around caretaking activities. These patterns of turn-taking sequences have been seen as the precursors of conversational turns.

Eye gaze and shared attention

Newborn infants are able to see and aim their gaze. This, together with basic orienting movements, are the first things that can be used to measure infant attention. Attention signals that the infant is ready to be receptive to communication, and it is mutual attention which is the basic necessity for successful communication.

By 4 months infants show a preference to visual stimuli that are coordinated with sound, suggesting the ability to coordinate visual and auditory information. Voluntary control of head and neck posture is also achieved so that in the period 3—6 months of age, orientation of the head and gaze are the signals that the infant is ready to communicate. When all visual contact is terminated this is perceived by the partner as withdrawal from communication.

Gesture

Initially a limited range of movements is available to the infant, and the same repertoire is used in a stereotyped way in different situations, before more appropriate differentiated motor responses develop for different contexts. Gestures, however, indicate communicative intention and as such they are specific motor acts. It has been suggested that adults facilitate the development of gestures by their repeated recognition and reinforcement of those specific motor acts which can be interpreted as conventional gestures.

Pointing is one of the most important preverbal gestures (Martlew, 1987), and it may be observed in the first few months when its function appears to be exploratory. At about 9 months it is used in conjunction with eye gaze to draw the mother into a communicative situation; it may be considered as a motor precursor to naming. Bates et al. (1979) found it to be the strongest predictor of language development in 9- to 18-month-old infants. It is usually a stable part of the communicative repertoire between 12 and 14 months.

Transition from preverbal to verbal communication

Protowords are those vocal phenomena which occur between babbling and conventional words. They have a limited range of expressive functions: approval, disapproval, wanting and rejecting. At about 14 months, protowords are used with gestures and predominate until about 19 months when they are superseded by single-word utterances, also accompanied by gestures (Martlew, 1987). By 20 months of age, most children have a considerable communicative repertoire which includes vocal, verbal and non-verbal acts. This is an important perspective when considering the language-impaired child and the paucity of communication that will be available to her or him.

This overview of prelinguistic development should serve to emphasise the vital contribution it makes to the child's language development. The interaction between environmental aspects and the development of maturity within the central nervous system (as in the use of vision, hearing and motor skills) is emphasised. However, suggestions that the language-impaired child's only problem is a failure to produce words in sufficient quantity or in the prescribed order is likely to be an oversimplification. Many other prerequisite skills are necessary before the child becomes verbal and all of them are vital to eventual communicative competence. The importance of the prelinguistic stage of development and competence in non-verbal skills to the management of the language-impaired child will be discussed in Chapter 4.

The second fact which is important to our understanding of language-impaired children is that for most children the development of language, the most complex cognitive skill of which the human race is capable, proceeds without any undue difficulty, so that by the age of 5 years old the child has mastered the major building blocks of the system. From the age of 5 the rest of childhood is spent refining and integrating the system so that language can be used for an increasingly complex range of tasks (reading, writing, debating, arguing, hypothesising, being factual or artistic or for fantasising etc). This fact is important for two reasons. First it emphasises the importance placed by society on competent verbal communication. In an age in which social value is measured by success, one of the major failures is an inability to communicate efficiently and effectively using verbal language. Adults who cannot do so immediately face a narrower range of life choices in terms of further education, employment and social integration; these adults become marginalised and isolated. So also does the child who is having difficulty mastering language skills. The British education system places great emphasis on language competence and the child who has difficulty with language acquisition loses out on educational opportunities and becomes socially isolated. Within the family, pressure also increases as a result of the social stigma of handicap and the frustration of trying to cope with a communication-impaired individual.

The importance of language competence within our society cannot be sufficiently emphasised. It is therefore vital that we gain a better understanding of how language acquisition proceeds in order to help language-handicapped individuals function effectively. Language impairment is not just of minor significance to the developing child; it is of major significance to the potential development of a complete, healthy and confident human being.

Secondly, if the major part of language acquisition is completed in the first 5 years of life and all subsequent gains are the complex integration of this basic skill, it suggests that a model of language processing, which is based solely on the normal adult, is a false perspective. The normal 5-year-old child and the process by which this stage of development is achieved have just as much to contribute to our knowledge of language processes as those models which are in more general use – these latter are based on the mature adult's response to cerebral dysfunction, usually as a result of lesions of the cerebral cortex. Even in the field of childhood language problems, the adult model involving lesions is the one that usually underlies most discussions of language processing or language impairment.

It has only recently been that those specifically interested in the study of childhood language problems from the child's perspective have come together to ask questions that could lead to a better integrated model for our understanding of language skill. Bishop and Mogford (1988) provide a good example of this in their work on *Language Development in Exceptional Circumstances*. After discussing the way in which language acquisition usually proceeds, they go on to ask five questions about language development which are important if we are to develop a more balanced model. These questions are then related to studies of language development in various groups including those whose environmental circumstances could be interrupting language development, those with sensory problems, those with structural abnormalities and those with cerebral dysfunction. This view of language development also emphasises the fact that even the most language-impaired individual has some communicative skill, however limited (and it may be very limited). This is a positive view of language difficulty which does not seek to 'write off' all those who do not achieve an imposed adult standard. It also emphasises the way in which the child is an active partner in determining his or her own progress with language development and not just a passive being which the adult shapes and influences.

Although the view that the child is active in communication from very early days has been current in our understanding for several decades, it has had little impact, until recently, on the way we manage developmental problems. The tendency to 'treat' the child, or in some way 'manage' the condition by imposing a predetermined standard model on the child, is still the most common view in language remediation techniques. If we allow ourselves to glimpse the possibility of being an active partner with the child in the process of language acquisition, therapy might take on a whole new perspective.

The Epidemiology of Language Problems in Children

The number of children at risk of developing language problems is important to our understanding of children's needs. Recent studies of the prevalence of language delay give an incidence of between 3% and 15%. These studies suffer from the fact that there is no real agreement about where the distinction between delayed and normal language development should be drawn. Three longitudinal studies, which considered both the prevalence of language difficulty and the evolution of the problems, were the Waltham Forest study (Stevenson and Richman, 1976), the Newcastle study (Fundudis, Kolvin and Garside, 1979), and the Dunedin study (Silva, McGee and Williams, 1983). There is a marked similarity between the methodology and results of these three studies. The children in all the studies were first assessed at the age of 3 years, and followed up at between 7 and 8 years of age. They all reported test data results from the WISC (Wechsler, 1974) and reading tests.

Although these studies were carried out in different locations using different definitions of language delay and slightly different measures of ability, results were similar. Early language delay was strongly predictive of low IQ and later reading difficulties. There was an association between language delay and later behavioural problems. None of these statements will come as a great surprise to experienced clinicians who will be familiar with the wide range of learning difficulties which are the frequent sequelae of 'late talking'.

Between 3% and 7.6% of the children in the three studies were identified as being language delayed. Stevenson (1984) suggested that, according to the Dunedin results, a prevalence of 7–8% of preschool children should be estimated. The criteria given for this figure were based on the Reynell Developmental Language Scales (Reynell, 1977) with the 5th centile as the cut-off point.

These data suggest a significant group of children who are 'at risk' for language development to be delayed. We need to consider what factors might influence a child's development and therefore contribute to or underlie a tendency to delayed language development. These factors are the subject of hypothesis rather than fact. It seems reasonable to suppose that there are certain fundamental requirements for language acquisition. These would be:

1. An ability to hear spoken language: if the child's environment contained

no spoken language or the child was unable to hear any then we might suppose that he or she would not learn any.

2. An environment in which language was spoken by competent speakers in a variety of communicative situations. It is clear that language is a complex skill and therefore competence might be related to an appreciation of those complexities; this means that the child needs to learn the skill from competent and creative speakers. We shall call these two requirements 'factors affecting language input'.

3. An ability to process the language heard and the context in which it takes place in order to 'make sense of it all': the complexity of the skill further suggests that a complex internal mechanism which will integrate all this experience is required. We shall call this requirement 'factors affecting language processing'.

4. An ability to form the units of spoken language with the organs of speech so they can be understood by others. The child needs to be able to produce the same code her- or himself in order to take part in the communicative exchange. We shall call this requirement 'factors affecting language output'.

It becomes clear, from observing children in a range of ordinary and clinical circumstances and from research studies, that the way in which these requirements interact and impinge on the individual differs widely. Even within one well-defined syndrome the range may be wide. This is probably a product of the infinite variety of human development. Nevertheless, the range of causal factors usually considered to be associated with language delay are usually summarised as affecting language input, processing or output as follows:

1. Factors affecting language input:
   (a) environmental factors: (i) social circumstances and (ii) bilingualism;
   (b) sensory deprivation: (i) hearing loss and (ii) visual problems.
2. Factors affecting language processing:
   (a) general cognitive deficiencies (mental handicap);
   (b) specific affective deficiencies (autism);
   (c) specific language deficiencies.
3. Factors affecting language output:
   (a) disorders of oromotor control;
   (b) structural abnormalities.

The way in which each of these might affect language development is not clearly understood. It is certainly not a simple matter of one clear cause having one defined effect. Indeed research studies have demonstrated that a wide range of possible outcomes might result from what, on the surface, look like similar factors influencing input, processing or output. It is well recognised that the range of language skills seen in a population of individuals with learning difficulties/mental handicap is very wide. Recently, attempts have been made to distinguish language subtypes for certain syndromes which affect general cognitive development, such as Down's syndrome (Rondal, 1988) and William's syndrome (Bellugi et al., 1988) among others. Others have addressed the wide range of ways in which input factors related to the child's environment and output factors related to the structure of the oral mechanism affect the child's language development. This research is well summarised by Mogford and Bishop (1988), who conclude that we are still a considerable way from understanding the factors that influence language development and from discovering the cause(s) of language impairment in children. They support the view that an interaction of factors may underlie difficulty with language development saying that 'Factors which on their own have no impact on language development might assume significance in combination' (p. 260). It is this combination effect which needs to be the focus of future research.

Deviant/Disordered Language Development

Whilst we can agree that the features of disordered language are present at some stage in normal language development, this does not seem to be sufficient reason to continue to call all types and degrees of language impairment 'language delay'. The very word 'delay' in fact suggests a belief that the child will somehow 'catch up'. Whilst Bishop and Edmundson (1987) showed that this was true for the majority of children they studied, there was still a group who had a persistent deficit, as described in Case 2. Similarly, where children do continue to have a large mismatch between aspects of their language and other skills, they can hardly be said to be the equivalent to the development of a normal younger child.

It is not that unusual for a child over the age of 10 years to present for initial assessment. As always it is important to review the preceding history of the situation and particularly to try to establish how the child's language abilities compares with other general learning abilities and social skills. This may reveal a situation in which a profile of the child's learning abilities extends over a wide range. Some general learning abilities might be in the normal range, with a slight delay evident in social skills, but with language skills showing a marked discrepancy. Further analysis might confirm that, for example, phonological development was mismatched in relation to syntactic or semantic skills. Speed of auditory verbal processing and word finding might be slow.

To describe such a child as language delayed fails to demonstrate the complexity of these problems. It also suggests that there was still time to catch up. A label of 'language delay' also fails to recognise the diverse nature of a child's strengths and needs, with some skills being well developed and others woefully inadequate. No normal developmental pattern would produce a pattern like this.

It is also relevant to introduce here the fact that some children lose language skills in childhood after a period of normal or near normal language development. This group of language-impaired children may be less commonly seen by general speech therapists, but this does not mean that they, or their problems, are not significant. Children with acquired aphasia will be discussed thoroughly in Chapter 9. They are mentioned here because they do demonstrate patterns of deviant language which, because they are acquired problems, cannot just be described as delayed.

The way in which congenital or neonatal cerebral lesions affect language development also suggests that language delay is not an appropriate term for this group either. Whilst it has long been recognised that a lesion in certain areas of the left cerebral hemisphere leads to language disturbance when this occurs in the adult, the effect of similar lesions before birth is not so clearly accepted. Lesions of Broca's and Wernicke's areas (in the left frontal lobe and left temporal lobe respectively) have been related to specific patterns of aphasia in adults (Broca's and Wernicke's aphasia). It has been suggested that in the infant a certain amount of reorganisation of brain function is possible. When a lesion occurs in Broca's or Wernicke's area before the first year of life, the right hemisphere takes over language specialisation, the role the damaged left hemisphere is no longer able to take (Bishop, 1988). However, there seem to be exceptions to most proposals about language development and cases in which early brain lesions in the left hemisphere underlie language disorder do occur as the example of Case 3 confirms.

Case 3

This boy was born at 34 weeks' gestation, the second child of two healthy, unrelated parents. At 29 weeks of pregnancy there was a small amount of bleeding, but monitoring at that stage did not give cause for further concern. His birth weight was 2.3 kg and he was considered rather small for dates. His parents began to be concerned when his motor development appeared rather different from his older, healthy and normally developing brother. At the age of 6 months a right hemiplegia was confirmed. He also had eczema but was otherwise well. A computed tomography (CT) scan of the brain showed that the left cerebral hemisphere was smaller than the right. There was an area of low density in the posterior part of the left frontal lobe in the region of Broca's area, and other smaller patches in the left temporal and parietal lobes suggestive of an old, left middle, cerebral artery infarct. With physiotherapy his motor skills improved and he walked independently at 26 months. However, at that stage he was not speaking, although his comprehension appeared good. Formal testing confirmed that it was within normal limits at age 2;6 years and continued to remain so throughout the period he received speech therapy. He was using a few vowel sounds to communicate as well as pointing and pulling.

A programme of therapy, which included the Makaton vocabulary, was introduced and he soon learned a useful number of signs. Despite his hemiplegia, he managed signing quite well and within 2 months was making up his own signs and linking signs accompanied by vowel sounds. He was over 3 years old before his first words developed. These were simple combinations of long vowels and glottal stops which had to be clarified by signing. Over the next year, he made good progress with communication and became more verbal as he mastered first velar and then bilabial nasals and plosives. Signing was still vital for intelligibility. He was admitted to a preschool language unit at age 4 years. By this stage his verbal language consisted of a wide vocabulary of open syllables in which the consonant–vowel combinations were predominantly plosives or nasals with long vowels and some glides. These were joined in short sequences of three or four words, often with glottal stops between each one. He continued to rely on signing for communication.

In this case it is clear that the normal sequence of sound acquisition has been disrupted resulting in a severe difficulty in communication through verbal language. Whilst it is not necessarily possible to say that all of this deficit is related to the early cerebral injury it has clearly been the major contributor, confirming that early lesions of the left cerebral hemisphere, and Broca's area, can have a considerable effect on language acquisition.

Despite this occasional confirmation of brain lesions, defining the group of children with deviant or disordered language is problematic. It is clear from the examples given so far that hindsight and the contribution of time to the evolution of the problem play a large part in our understanding. In trying to distinguish language disorder from delay, the medical model of diagnosis has made a major contribution. The traditional definitions and descriptions have a distinctly medical flavour about them, but have recently been widened to include terminology which owes its origins to psychology, linguistics and phonetics, as well as better defined clinical descriptions. Children with isolated impairment of language, with other skills being normal, but for whom none of the usual predisposing factors can be identified, have been said to have a specific language disorder (i.e. the problem is specific to language development). This definition has generally been arrived at by exclusion:

1. Not a hearing loss.
2. Not mental handicap.
3. Not due to the child's environment.
4. Not an emotional problem.
5. Therefore it must be a language disorder.

This simple model might seem quite appealing. It suggests that all that is required for understanding and diagnosing language disorder is gradually to eliminate other interfering factors. Language disorder is then the bit left over which cannot be explained. This is hardly satisfactory. Whilst some children may appear to have problems with a single origin, in the vast majority some or even all of these factors may have been or are present. This suggests that it is an interaction effect of the previously identified factors in each individual case which leads to the particular clinical problem. Advocates of this view have suggested a multifactorial aetiology of language disorder where language impairment is the final common pathway for a number of factors which interrupt development (Bishop, 1987).

If we take a multifactorial view of the aetiology of language disorder, we arrive at a definition of the problems which is rather more positive because it is a definition by inclusion. It recognises the contribution which is made by both extrinsic and intrinsic factors to the child's development as in the following definition:

> A language disorder is that language profile which, although it may be associated with a history of hearing, learning, environmental and emotional difficulties, cannot be attributed to any one of these alone, or even just the sum of these effects, and in which one or more of the following is also seen:
>
> 1. A close positive family history of specific difficulty in language development.
> 2. Evidence of cerebral dysfunction, either during development or by the presence of neurological signs.
> 3. A mismatch between the various subsystems of language in relation to other aspects of cognitive development.
> 4. A failure to catch up these differences with 'generalised' language help.

The familial aspects of language disorder have been discussed by Robinson (1987). The excess of boys presenting with the condition (Robinson gives a ratio of 3.8:1) also points towards a genetic connection. However, apart from a number of syndromes in which language disorder may also occur (see Appendix I), it has not yet proved possible to isolate a specific genetic marker for language disorder. That specific language problems are related to cerebral dysfunction, particularly lesions of the cerebral cortex, has been the major discussion of language impairment in adults. Whilst it must not be overlooked in children, evidence for clear cerebral lesions in children with developmental language disorders is very rare. For those presenting with acquired disorders, the presence of unilateral cerebral lesions is significant in one subgroup (see Chapter 9). However, some children who present with developmental language disorders do so against a background of information that indicates some cerebral dysfunction of which epilepsy is the most common marker (Robinson cites 21% of his Moorhouse School sample with definite seizures and a further 11% with possible seizures). Other signs of unusual neurological development include the higher degree of clumsiness associated with motor incompetence (up to 90% according to Robinson) and anomalous cerebral dominance as demonstrated by the higher proportion of children who are left- or mixed-handed. The mismatch between language development and other aspects of cognitive development has already been mentioned, as has the importance of time in understanding the disorder. However, the latter is not an excuse for not taking action. The fact, previously mentioned, of the usual pattern of language acquisition being complete by the age of 5 years is in itself part of the argument which says that intervention in language disorder should take place early in order to ensure that the maximum potential is reached in accordance with the general developmental trend, rather than an approach which advocates waiting to see how bad it becomes before taking any action. The first course of action for a child who presents with 'late talking' is often to provide more language learning experiences. It is when this 'more of the same' approach fails to close the gaps in development that a further sign of a more persistent developmental deviancy becomes clear.

This definition is illustrated by the following two case histories (in addition to Cases 2 and 3 already presented).

Case 4

This boy was 3 years old when seen for assessment. His mother, a single parent, was concerned that he 'didn't seem to talk at all'. He was the second healthy child from two healthy, unrelated parents, who had recently been divorced. There was a history of two pregnancies which had ended in miscarriages between the two live births. The other child was a boy, 7 years older, who was described as well and developing normally. There was no known family history of language difficulties on the mother's side of the family. However, it was difficult to establish if this was also true for the boy's father, who had been adopted at the age of 3 years; there was some suggestion that he may also have been a late talker. The boy had been described as 'small for dates' at birth (i.e. on the light side for gestational age). He had been induced 4 weeks early and delivered by emergency caesarean section with a birth weight of 2 lb and 4 oz (1.12 kg). He spent a month in the special care baby unit and was nasogastrically fed. He was late in developing the ability to suck and had much greater difficulty with chewing. He would only tolerate soft and mashed foods and was often known to choke and vomit anything with lumps. He was reported to have said 'daddy' at the age of 2 years, but that was the only word he had ever been heard to say.

Even as a baby he had been described as quiet and did not progress to babbling. When seen for initial assessment he was making a small number of high pitched sounds and using a few gestures to communicate, which he had learned over the previous 3 months. Otherwise he tended to point and grunt to make his needs known. He was described as often frustrated by his difficulty in communicating, such that temper tantrums were frequent. This had become particularly noticeable in the preceding 6 weeks, since he had started attending a preschool playgroup for four mornings a week.

On assessment his play skills were within the normal range for his age. However, his verbal comprehension was rather lower, at around the 2;3 year level. He did not dribble but was not keen to imitate mouth movements or sounds. He did point at objects he wanted to play with and used a few gestures with his mother. A physical examination by the paediatric neurologist indicated a mild bilateral motor disorder, with a mild tremor in the upper limbs and very brisk reflexes. He was also mildly unsteady on his feet, not well organised when attempting to catch or kick a ball, and clumsy in fine motor movements such as piling up bricks or playing with a posting box.

Case 5

Another boy, also referred at 3 years of age, was the only child of a single parent family in which the mother had always been the sole caretaker. His mother was able to give little in terms of detail about his early development, but he was born by normal delivery after a normal full-term pregnancy with a birth weight around 7 lb (3.15 kg). He had been a healthy and lively baby who fed well. Other aspects of his development had proceeded normally. At the age of 1 year he had a febrile convulsion lasting 10 minutes. He had been seen at home by his GP but not hospitalised; there had been no further evidence of epilepsy. He had said his first words at 9 months and had gradually acquired a range of single words over the next year. However, he had failed to progress to joining words as expected, having only recently started to do so. He tended to echo the last words of sentences said to him and his mother felt his understanding was poor. He knew a number of body parts and could point to them on request. However, he was unable to carry out simple commands like 'put teddy on the chair'. It was difficult to sustain his attention for a task with an unknown adult. He would play quietly with his mother but in a manner more suited to a younger child. He would name pictures of objects in a book and all single words were intelligible. Physical examination was unremarkable. A hearing test suggested a mild conductive loss, but this was not thought sufficient to affect speech development. Indeed, the fact that his single words were clearly articulate suggests that he had at least sufficient hearing for the rudiments of verbal language.

Both of these cases include examples of the different factors thought to influence language development. In the first, there is a history of a stormy neonatal period and clear evidence of early problems in motor development, both in oral function and more generally. In the second, the neonatal period seems to have proceeded normally with only one febrile convulsion at the end of the first year to suggest any cerebral dysfunction. In both cases it was difficult to establish the family history, as is often the case, but history may have been a factor in Case 4 at least. Both boys had demonstrated some good developmental abilities, and equally both had made some progress with communication skills, such that they could communicate in a limited way with their main caretaker. The inclusive definition of language development, with an holistic view of the child, his or her environment, history and progress, allows us to suggest that both of these children present with language disorders and that a number of factors had contributed to their present manifestation.

Receptive–expressive continuum

These case histories also demonstrate something of the heterogeneous nature of language disorder. It is not a unitary condition, and that is not just because we might expect to find some variation between children. Rather the language profiles seem to suggest that different aspects of the language system might be differentially affected. In the grossest sense this can be referred to as a continuum from predominantly receptive language difficulty to predominantly expressive difficulty. Whilst some children might be placed at the extreme ends of this continuum, most will have a mixed pattern (i.e. problems in both receptive and expressive language as in both of these cases, although Case 4, like Case 3, suggests a greater expressive problem).

The major problem with this description of language disorder is its very subjective nature. There are no 'landmarks' along the continuum to help us make cross-child comparisons or define related groups of problems. It is also true that, because expressive language is the outward manifestation of the problem, we are all aware of cases in clinical practice in which receptive problems have been overlooked. This has led to the situation where diagnosis using this continuum has often been weighted towards the expressive end. The term 'receptive dysphasia' has been used in the literature for children with one pattern of language disorder; however, it is not always used consistently. Some research studies that have used it applied it to groups of children in whom the problem appeared to be predominantly expressive, according to the clinical descriptions given (Rutter, 1978b). However the receptive–expressive continuum is a helpful place to begin when diagnosing language disorder, provided careful clinical descriptions are used which are then consistently applied.

The Development of Terminology for Language Disorder

Developing a consistent terminology from clinical description in the field of language disorder has involved many disciplines. The converging influences of medicine, linguistics and psychology has led to an expansion of the terminology. Whilst no universally agreed classification is in use, a distinction does arise between a medical approach to classification and its terminology and a linguistic approach and the terminology it uses. Bishop and Rosenbloom (1987) suggest that diagnostic labels arising from medical terminology in language disorder seem to have three purposes: the description of observed clinical symptoms, an indication of the underlying mechanism or an indication of aetiology. Thus, for example, hearing loss may be an underlying mechanism to language impairment of which otitis media is the aetiology and in which unintelligible speech is the observed symptom.

A linguistic approach to the classification of language disorder would include terms indicating at what level the language system had broken down (i.e. phonology, grammar, semantics or pragmatics), whether this was a receptive or expressive problem and whether it was immature or deviant. Thus, unintelligible speech could be described as a breakdown at the phonological level at which expressive language was either immature (containing evidence of processes generally used by younger children as in Case 1) or deviant (such that the processes were highly unusual and not usually seen in the processes of normal language development, as in Case 3). They go on to suggest a two-way classification of language disorders which combines the best of both of these systems. Such a combined approach aims to enlarge upon the useful features of each so as to reflect more accurately clinical presentation. It is an advantage to use such a descriptive system when working in a multidisciplinary team, when clarity between different professionals is required.

It is always important to remember why particular terminology has been adopted and from what perspective. As more disciplines converge on the study of language impairment in childhood, a wider range of possibilities is opened up. The purpose of using particular terminology might be:

1. To allow discussion across disciplines.
2. To differentiate specific types of disorders or syndromes.

Defining Language Disorder Syndromes

The definition of syndromes is a common medical/clinical exercise. If it acts as a way of clarifying a complex clinical situation, it can be very helpful. The present proliferation in terminology of language disorder has not always been so helpful; whilst it aims for clarity in what we are talking about, it most often has the opposite effect. We find ourselves talking at cross-purposes because another professional uses terminology we may have abandoned as old-fashioned or out of date (commonly the case when some continue to use the term 'developmental dysphasia', which we must surely move away from) or, more usually, because we have all interpreted the terminology from a slightly different clinical perspective (as with the term semantic–pragmatic disorder, now in common clinical use – see below). The purpose of defining language disorder syndromes is:

1. To outline natural history and substantiate prognosis.
2. To allocate appropriate treatment/management.
3. To enable appropriate comparisons between children.
4. To facilitate research.

The terminology used to define language disorder syndromes will largely be determined by the theoretical model(s) adopted. Because of the long-standing influence of the 'lesionist' in the study of language impairment, the adult model of specific lesions resulting in particular language disorder syndromes still impinges on the study of language problems in children. This, in part, accounts for the continued popularity of the term 'developmental dysphasia' – the term is surely nonsense, for how can we use a term which describes the loss of a skill to label one which has never been acquired in the first place. The continued use of this label reinforces the use of the adult-based model, rather than encouraging the development of models appropriate for childhood language problems. Equally, attempts to draw direct relationships between the language problems described after cerebral lesions in adults and those seen in developmental language disorder have not been productive. Also the adult syndromes have not been particularly useful when describing the features of language impairment seen in acquired childhood aphasia (Lees, 1989). It has been suggested that they are only of limited use in the study of adult aphasia anyway (Marshall, 1986).

Recent attempts, by Rapin and Allen (1987), to define a range of language disorder syndromes in children have met with some success, although they have yet to be rigorously assessed. Their definitions borrowed terminology from medicine and linguistics, and they tried to cover the range from predominantly receptive to predominantly expressive disorders by describing the six following different language disorder syndromes.

Verbal auditory agnosia

This is also called word deafness. There is no comprehension in the auditory—verbal channel and the child is unable to understand anything that is said to him or her. In the initial stages of this disorder, the child is often thought to be deaf but a hearing test should confirm normal hearing. It can be a severely handicapping disorder with a poor prognosis in which alternative communication (usually a sign system) remains vital for comprehension of language.

Semantic—pragmatic deficit

Fluent, well-formed speech is characterised by early echolalia and later delayed echolalia in which the child just repeats what is said or replaces conversation with long monologues of learned speech (often from television advertisements). This is an indication of the child's underlying difficulty with verbal comprehension which is usually literal. The child often responds to key words rather than to the whole meaning of a sentence. Where expressive language is not echolalic it is often made up of short, predictable and over-used phrases so that language lacks any creative quality. These phrases are referred to as verbal stereotypes. Perseverations also occur, which is the tendency to use the same verbal expression again and again without any realisation of its appropriateness. Circumlocution, the tendency to talk around the subject in a vaguely related manner but without specific content, is another feature. This disorder can also be a very persistent condition. The older child is likely to continue to comprehend literally and use stereotyped and empty language to communicate.

Lexical–syntactic deficit

The major feature is a severe word retrieval difficulty. The child seems to know what he or she wants to say but is unable to select the appropriate word to do so. There is usually some difficulty forming connected utterances and comprehending grammar. When unable to name accurately, some naming errors may occur in which non-words close to the target word replace the intended item. These are called paraphasias and are of three main types: semantic paraphasias where the item is related in meaning to the target (e.g. chair replaces table), phonemic paraphasias in which the item is related in sound to the intended target (thrimble replaces thimble) and neologisms (literally nonsense words) in which it is not possible to discern the target. In addition, the child may employ other strategies to overcome the word-finding problem including the use of a gestural replacement or the use of a more general word or term like 'thing'. Although it can be a severe problem, it usually becomes less evident in the older child who can learn to cope with it by generating self-cueing strategies or by simply changing the subject.

Phonological–syntactic deficit

These children are dysfluent, speak in short utterances and often make errors which are termed 'morphological' (confusing tense markings, plural and other grammatical markers and the omission of small words called functors). Comprehension of these items may also be impaired but less than expression. Phonological contrasts are reduced so that speech is also unintelligible, but usually immature rather than deviant. Older children may continue to have some trouble with complex grammatical rules, particularly in written language.

Phonological programming deficit

Here the length of utterances is longer, but unintelligibility of the speech is a moderate to severe problem. There is probably a receptive component to the processing of speech–sound information in this disorder, but it is poorly understood. Speech–sound contrasts are considerably reduced but unlikely to be deviant.

Verbal dyspraxia

Speech is markedly dysfluent and severely unintelligible. Comprehension is usually adequate. Expressive language is confined to a few sounds or at best short utterances. There is often evidence of motor planning deficit and possibly other motor deficits as well. These children may become very frustrated and, in severe cases, may require the long-term use of an alternative communication system (usually signing).

Rapin and Allen (1987) discussed their use of these subtypes to diagnose the language difficulties in 126 preschool children. In this initial communication, there were only four severely disordered autistic children who could not be assigned to one of the language subtypes. However, they are still in the process of reporting a larger group. Using the definitions of these six syndromes in clinical practice has proved useful in providing a common basis for the various professionals involved in the diagnosis of language disorder. However, it has also raised several, as yet unanswered questions. Whilst some children, such as Cases 3 and 4 seem to fit one of the syndromes quite well (Case 3: verbal dyspraxia; Case 4: semantic–pragmatic deficit), others seem to have more pervasive disorders which cover a wider range of symptoms (Case 2). Equally, some children seem to have a pattern of language disorder which changes as the problem evolves. Whilst this is more obvious in acquired childhood aphasia, it can also be seen in some developmental problems. What looks like a predominantly phonological problem can, after the phonological system has matured, appear to mask a word-finding problem, for example. Further use of this type of classification within a clinical setting is required to evaluate its usefulness. However, it does begin to provide a useful framework within which the range of expressive and receptive language problems observed in children can be set, in order that we can begin to discuss the severity and prognosis of such conditions. It has also been used as the basis for an expert system for the differential diagnosis of language disorder which will be discussed in Chapter 3 (Dalton, 1989).

The Clinical Dilemma

Let us return to the clinical dilemma so well defined by Coombes (1987), because this is the basis of this book. 'How to know what to do' is influenced by two factors: a theoretical model and thorough assessment of the presenting situation. Chapter 2 sets out to discuss the question of appropriate clinical assessment of children's language. After discussing possible assessment procedures, the process of differential diagnosis within the clinical setting is considered in more detail in Chapter 3. Once the problem has been comprehensively described, knowing 'what to do', including the who and the where, is discussed in Chapters 4, 5 and 6. Appropriate therapy and management practices for language-impaired children are set out and discussed. These chapters also tackle the questions of when to do whatever is required, and, equally importantly, 'when to stop' (Coombes, 1987). However, it must be clear from this initial chapter that our understanding of language disorder is always growing and changing. It is therefore important to continue to remember the place of effective clinical research in working with language-disordered children, which is considered in Chapter 8.

Chapter 2
Formal and Informal Assessment

Summary

The assessment procedure is approached from the child's perspective and what he or she needs to know about language. A wide selection of formal tests and developmental checklists is reviewed as a starting point for busy clinicians who wish to make informed and appropriate choices. Informal assessment techniques and materials are discussed and the aim is to describe a language environment in which the child can function, in order to replicate that in therapy.

This chapter deals with how the appropriate information required in order to manage a language-disordered child might be gathered. Whilst all clinicians continue to develop individual assessment techniques and ways of looking at children, standardised assessments obviously have a place. The pattern of difficulties and the interpretation of responses and results can confirm and focus general clinical observations; however, therapists should not feel pressurised into providing 'test scores' alone, because they give minimal information about the child, what the child needs to know about language and what the child can do with the language he or she has. A detailed report of careful observations in several situations may be just as appropriate for co-workers, and although there may be some controversy as to whether to use a formal or informal approach, for most of us the aim is to achieve a workable balance.

Approaches to Formal Assessment

This section is not intended to be a detailed, descriptive list of tests, because there have been several extensive reviews in the literature (Bishop and Mogford, 1988), which help in the tracking down of a test that seems to cover just the area needed to quantify a particular child's problem. Unfortunately, feelings of relief may give way to those of uncertainty on being faced with a wide choice of assessment possibilities.

Time limits and availability will drastically reduce the final number of tests that the therapist can gather and use and it therefore becomes very important to make the right choice. A new test may be an interesting prospect, well packaged and by a well-known author, but it may not be better than others previously published. The test material and manual will require careful examination to determine whether they will answer the questions being asked. For example, one of the most frequent reasons for using a standardised test is to produce a comparison with the child's peers. Since many tests originate in the USA, vocabulary and cultural differences often limit the usefulness of such a comparison. Equally it would be reasonable to expect that a high number of subjects from a wide range of socioeconomic backgrounds had been involved in the standardisation of any test, and such details should be given in the manual. It may then come as a surprise to find that a test you thought applied to the 'general' population was in fact standardised on 20 children from the same socioeconomic background (Carrow, 1974). Interpreting the results in this context would need to be done cautiously, and it may be one of the reasons for deciding not to use a particular test.

Formal assessments should fulfil two further basic requirements: they should be easy to administer and score (if not, an examiners' course should be mandatory) and the test materials should be appealing. Given that these factors are so essential, it is amazing that tests continue to fail these basic requirements. Perhaps it is difficult to fit children to psychometric procedures, or is it the other way round?

Scoring and statistics

The majority of standard assessments record quantitative results. Usually scoring is based on a pass/fail system, and the examiner has to rely on descriptive notes made during the test to make any further qualitative judgements about the child's pattern of response. Thus, two children who gain the same test score may be clinically very different. For example, the Test for Reception of Grammar (Bishop, 1983) contains 20 sections, called blocks. Two children aged 5 years who both pass six blocks (i.e. they obtain a raw score of 6) would be assessed as having a similar comprehension level. However, a comparison of the test sheet could show that one child passed the first six blocks and then failed to pass any subsequent blocks, whilst the other child passed the first two blocks, failed the third, passed the fourth, failed the fifth and passed the next three blocks, and then failed to pass any others. To gain a better understanding of the second child's performance a closer analysis is necessary.

In a more extreme example, one child may completely ignore the test procedure and another may narrowly miss success by omitting a small element from the required response. The children's scores may be statistically significant in terms of standard deviation from the mean, but other factors, such as rate of progress over time, response to the testing situation and the pattern of those responses, will be important in determining the clinical significance of the results (Muller, 1984). The whole point about assessment is surely to determine when and how the child is failing, and then how to help him or her to succeed. Standardised assessments, by sampling a small part of the child's behaviour, can only help pinpoint certain difficulties and perhaps determine how the child functions in relation to his or her peer group.

In summary, it would be important to ask the following questions.

1. Is the test appealing and well designed?
2. Is the manual informative about test procedure?
3. Is the scoring straightforward?
4. Will the test suit the particular child in question?
5. Will it yield all the information required?

To avoid the disappointment of finding that a test is totally inappropriate, it may be useful to ask other colleagues and co-workers for their views on new developments. There is usually someone local who will give an 'off the cuff' critique, or the loan of a manual. In theory then, clinicians have, at their disposal, a wealth of standardised assessment material, but after due consideration the final choice may be one robust test which fulfils the criteria listed above, coupled with several useful smaller tests, or subtests of other assessments.

Assessments for Speech and Language-impaired Children

This section, based on personal clinical experience, is a discussion and evaluation of various assessments, some which are standardised and others which are more informal but follow developmental guidelines.

The Reynell Developmental Language Scales (Revised) (RDLS)

Probably the most popular test in use by speech therapists in this country is the RDLS (Reynell, 1977, revised 1985; McMillen, Mule and Lees, 1987). Although it is sometimes felt to be rather lengthy, the comprehension section can be fun and is popular with many children despite its shortcomings, because the child may help with setting up and putting away the various toys. There is a lot of change and movement to encourage interest, except for the highly distractible for whom standardised assessment would be inappropriate. The section dealing with colour, number, length and preposition together is rather overloaded, especially for language-disordered children. It is often difficult to tell precisely what the errors should be attributed to. However, overall the comprehension section does give an accurate picture of areas of difficulty and where to begin when planning treatment. It is well researched and standardised on British children. Given the variety of test material, it is a shame that the score system, like so many others, is pass/fail. The failure to take account of many children's needs for a repetition of instructions is another limitation.

The test is of little value for the child with very poor attention control (level 1–2) (see under 'The Wolfson assessment'). Such a child would be unlikely to get past the large toy section and this would not be an accurate reflection of his or her comprehension skills. It really would be unlikely to reveal anything not already known about the child, i.e. that he or she had poor attention! In such a case, a more informal approach, or perhaps the Symbolic Play Test (Lowe and Costello, 1976; see below), should be considered.

Many clinicians find the expressive section of the test difficult to score, although the revised manual is much more explicit about this. It is not clear what the various subtests are sampling, and many people use the comprehension section and use other tests for expressive language.

The Symbolic Play Test (SPT)

The SPT (Lowe and Costello, 1976) is an appealing, short assessment. The detailed and standardised checklist of behaviours, coupled with a variety of small toy play situations, can give a useful insight into the young, language-impaired child's 'language readiness'. Little or no verbal guidance is given during the test, and some children find this daunting, but it can work to the advantage of the child with poor attention. It is reasonable for the examiner to touch the test material in order to encourage the child to do so. However, very young children are rarely concerned about this, since they are used to playing alongside their friends rather than with them. Because of the limited verbal interaction required, it can be useful for the timid child. It would be interesting to see if further developments were possible in line with this type of test. Information about conceptual/symbolic/sequencing development is valuable in the language-impaired child, and additional or optional toys might widen the range of appeal of the test. What do you do if the child is uninspired by a doll or a tractor and would prefer a spaceship or a pony?

Renfrew tests

The Word Finding Vocabulary Test (Renfrew, 1972c)

This test of confrontational naming was designed for children aged 3–8 years. It consists of 59 items which are black and white line drawings on separate cards. The child is asked to name the pictures presented in test order; the response is noted, as is any tendency towards hesitation, overt searching behaviour, self-correction or no response. Equivalent age scores are available for both boys and girls.

The Action Picture Test (Renfrew, 1972a)

This test is very quick to administer. It contains ten pictures, all coloured line drawings, of people engaged in simple activities. The child is asked a number of simple questions which should elicit a sentence in response. The child's response is recorded and analysed according to the information contained in the sentence and grammatical accuracy. Age equivalent scores are available.

The Bus Story Test (Renfrew, 1972b)

Whilst the idea of this test is generally appealing, the content does not go down well with all children. A series of pictures in a book represent the activities of a naughty bus. The examiner tells the child the story according to a script and then asks the child to retell the story. The response is tape-recorded and transcribed. The sentences obtained are analysed for content and grammatical accuracy. It is one of the few tests available that considers the child's ability to use language in a connected narrative. It has been found to be highly predictive of persistent language difficulty (Bishop and Edmundson, 1987).

Taken together these three tests are quick to administer, easily portable and fairly appealing to children, although they have tended to go out of fashion in some quarters, particularly among professionals training speech therapy students. This is possibly due to the non-technical method used to assess grammar and information in the latter two. However, they are still useful clinical tools for the discriminating therapist.

Test for Reception of Grammar (TROG)

TROG (Bishop, 1983) is enjoyed by children. It is quick and the pictures are colourful and sometimes funny. The information yielded can be very useful in planning treatment, particularly for those who are 7, 8 or 9 years old and still having problems in high level grammatical skills. It is a test of the auditory–verbal comprehension of syntax, as was designed for use with language-disordered children aged 4–12 years. It consists of a picture book of 80 coloured line drawings, four to each A4-sized page. The items are grouped into 20 sections (or blocks), with four test sentences in each section, arranged in increasing complexity from single nouns to complex sentences. The examiner presents the test sentences verbally and the child responds by pointing to one of the four suggested pictures given for that item. Older children may respond by saying the number (1–4) of the chosen picture, and the number of the picture chosen is marked on the response form. The examiner may repeat the test sentence if necessary, and any hesitation or self-correction in the child's response may also be noted. The child must produce four correct responses in each section to be credited with understanding at that syntactic level. The pattern of errors can be analysed to indicate whether the child has a significant difficulty with certain grammatical structures (called G errors) or a more general comprehension difficulty related to the vocabulary (called L errors). There is a picture-pointing vocabulary test which allows the examiner to ensure that the child's errors are not just a reflection of poor word knowledge. The test results can be analysed according to age-equivalent scores or centile levels.

The Boehm Test of Basic Concepts

The revised Boehm test (Boehm, 1986), like its predecessor (Boehm, 1971), has been well researched. It is easy to administer to one child or even groups of children. For this reason it is sometimes included as part of a screening battery in primary or first schools where it could be useful to have a standardised test of concept development. However, despite recent revisions, the illustrations are not always clear or interesting (apart from a few minor alterations the art work has not been revised). For each section, detailed instructions on how to introduce the material and score the test items is given. In all subtests, children are provided with an answer booklet and asked to mark their response in pencil, e.g. 'Mark the star that is at the top'. More complex combinations include 'Mark the shortest flower that is between two tall flowers'. Concepts are divided into four basic categories: space, quantity, time and miscellaneous concepts; the whole test includes a total of 50 concepts. Other subsections added to the revised addition include antonyms, synonyms and a section in which concepts are used in combination. One important criticism of the test is its reliance on two-dimensional representation. Prepositional concepts do not translate well to two dimensions. A combination of two- *and* three-dimensional material could be a useful addition to the assessment of conceptual development.

The Bracken Basic Concept Scale (Bracken, 1984)

This is a short, visually interesting test of concept development for children aged 4–10 years. Instructions are delivered verbally, and the child is required to point to one of four pictures. It has 11 subtests covering colour, letter identification, numbers and counting, comparisons (same, equal and different) and shape. The subtotal scores of the first five subtests are then used to determine a child's school readiness composite (called

SRC) which, in turn, influences where the examiner begins on the next six subtests. For example, an SRC score of 0–10 would mean the examiner subsequently begins at the first stage, stage A, a score of 31–35 at stage F and 56–61 at the final stage, stage K. This cuts down the time the test takes and ensures that material is presented at a level appropriate to the child's ability. The last five sections, with examples from each stage, are given below.

Section 6
Direction and position: there are 55 test items. Stage A begins at item one, 'Which book is open', whilst stage K is item 55, 'Which people are walking in opposite directions'.

Section 7
Social and emotional: this has 29 items which include gender (man, boy, male, female), family (brother, sister) and feelings (happy, sick, curious, disappointed).

Section 8
Size: these 16 items range from big/little to deep/shallow and light/heavy.

Section 9
Texture and material: there are 24 items some of which are shiny, loud, dark, cold, solid, dull and loose.

Section 10
Time and sequences: there are 35 items which range from the first question, 'Which child has finished drinking', to the last one, 'What is always in the sky?'

The raw scores are converted to standard scores which can then be plotted on a summary profile. Thus the child can be compared to the peer group, although the norms are from the USA. The pattern of errors can also be analysed and areas of poor conceptual development identified. There is an optional language package which accompanies the test. This includes well-illustrated, colour picture material, stories and composite pictures which could be used when working with individuals or in groups once areas of difficulty have been established.

Carrow Elicited Language Inventory (CELI)

The CELI (Carrow, 1974) is an American test and, therefore, as far as the standardisation is concerned, it should be used with care. A further disadvantage is that the population used in its development was very small.

The test lacks interest and the onus is on the examiner to keep the child involved; however, the clinical information it yields can be very interesting. Given that language-disordered children do not always produce a great deal of expressive language, it is often difficult to determine if they have truly understood and generalised a particular grammatical construction and, perhaps more importantly, how they deal with and process incoming information. The pattern of responses and errors given on repetition can give the clinician a clue as to what the child is processing, e.g. does the child ignore negatives and/or embedded clauses? Does the child understand the passive construction?

The Test of Word Finding (German, 1986)

This test is a recent development in the assessment of word finding in children. Carefully researched, the model which underlies it is described by German (1989). It is based on four assumptions:

1. Children's word-finding skills can be evaluated in a task which requires them to find words in various formats and so puts demands on their retrieval system.
2. These skills can be observed when they are asked to name words in different syntactic and semantic categories.
3. These skills can be categorised according to accuracy, speed, response type and the presence of self-cueing strategies, such as gesture and other verbalisations.
4. The child's word knowledge needs to be established before any naming errors can really be considered as word-finding errors.

The test is suitable for children aged 6–12 years. It contains five naming sections: (1) naming pictures of nouns, (2) sentence completion naming, (3) description naming, (4) naming pictures of verbs and (5) naming pictures of categories. The child obtains an accuracy score for each section which is the number of correct names given on the first response. This can be converted to both percentile rank and standard score (the norms are from the USA and some of the vocabulary is exclusive). Responses are also timed and it is possible to identify items in which there was a significant delay in response time. Thus, both an accuracy and time profile can be obtained for each child to determine whether their naming was characteristically fast and accurate or slow and accurate, fast and inaccurate or slow and inaccurate. In order to differentiate word-finding errors from items that the child does not know, there is a word comprehension test. This covers all the items in the test and is completed by the child pointing to a series of pictures. The clear model on which this test is based, its appealing presentation and thorough analysis of assessment data makes this a valuable test for the assessment of word-finding difficulties in language-disordered children.

Porch Index of Communicative Ability in Children (PICAC)

Developed from a test for adults and following the same model, the PICAC (Porch, 1972) claims to measure basic communicative abilities in children aged 3–12 years. There are two scales, basic and advanced, which contain a number of subtests. These subtests consider communicative skills in five modalities: auditory, visual, verbal, gestural and graphic.

The graphic skills can be tested separately from the main body of the test if assessment time dictates such a need. The test material consists of ten common objects, some of which are more robust than others. The standard conditions of the test procedure are written out in full in the test booklet. One of the major contributions of this test is the multidimensional scoring scheme which is based on five aspects of the child's response: accuracy, responsiveness, completeness, promptness and efficiency. These aspects are combined in a 16-point scoring system. Whilst some examiners will consider this extreme, experience confirms that it does not take long to learn. Any disadvantages are soon outweighed by the advantages of being able to describe clearly a child's response, which is something that can easily be transferred beyond the boundaries of this test to clinical practice as a whole. It makes the whole process of observation a more active, accurate and objective procedure. The test results can be plotted on a range of graphs and percentile levels are also given for each subtest as well as each modality (the norms are from the USA).

Illinois Test of Psycholinguistic Abilities (ITPA)

The ITPA (Kirk, McCarthy and Kirk, 1968) is an in-depth assessment of many different aspects of language processing. It has been well researched and has been the subject of debate for 20 years. Initially hailed as an all encompassing language test for everything, it suffered an inevitable backlash during the 1970s. The theoretical framework which accompanies the ITPA may seem quite confusing at first glance. Essentially, the authors suggest that it is possible to isolate and measure discrete language and language-related skills. It presupposes that we receive information via auditory and visual channels (examined in auditory and visual reception subtests). This information is then compared, organised and integrated (called 'association', which is examined in both visual and auditory modes) for ready retrieval (called 'expression' and measured in manual and verbal modes). These are thought to be representational skills, involving conscious thought, reasoning etc. Other skills are thought to be automatic. These are defined as not requiring conscious thought or reasoning and include the recall of a series of digits (auditory memory and sequencing) and symbols (visual memory and sequencing), the knowledge of grammatical rules (the grammatical closure subtest), scanning and perceptual tasks (visual closure subtest) and the phonological characteristics of words (sound blending and auditory closure subtests).

The ITPA has been criticised for failing to prove the 'separateness' of these skills (Newcomer et al., 1973). Further criticism has been aimed at the heavy language load of the majority of the subtests (Smith and Marx, 1971). For example, the visual memory test looks at the subject's ability to sequence non-meaningful symbols. However, to score highly on this subtest, the subject will use language to label and give meaning to the symbols and thus remember more of them. In summary then the ITPA model is directly at odds with recent notions of cognition and language development, which are more interactive (Bloom and Lahey, 1978; Cooper, Moodley and Reynell, 1978; Udwin and Yule, 1983; Chiat and Hirson, 1987). However, the six representational subtests can provide some useful insights into the language-disordered child's ability to retrieve, organise and manipulate language, particularly in the school-aged child. These subtests are described below.

Auditory reception

The child is required to derive meaning from verbally presented material and give a yes/no response. There are 50 items. It is graded in difficulty beginning with easy items like 'Do dogs eat?' and going on to more complex ones like 'Do dials yawn?' and 'Do wingless birds soar?'.

Visual reception

This subtest is comparable to the auditory test but in the visual modality. There are 40 items for which a stimulus picture and 4 possible response pictures are provided. The child points in response to the instructions 'See this? Find one here' and has to find the object or situation which is conceptually similar.

Auditory association

This tests the child's ability to relate and manipulate concepts presented verbally. There are 42 items which are presented in the style: 'A dog has hair, a fish has....'. A range of correct and incorrect responses is given against which the child's response can be compared.

Visual association

This is a visual subtest similar in style to the preceding auditory one. The child is presented with one stimulus card and four optional response pictures, one of which is related to the stimulus. There are 20 items for which the question is 'What goes with this?'. At a basic level, this includes a sock which goes with a shoe and a hammer which goes with a nail. At a higher level, there are visual analogies for which the child is asked 'If this goes with this [two items are shown] then what goes with this?' (child's cue to respond by making the analogy).

Manual expression

There are 15 pictures of common objects and the child is asked to 'Show me what we do with a ....'. The child has to mime the response.

Verbal expression

This assesses the child's ability to express advanced concepts verbally. There are five items, and the child is presented with one familiar object at a time (e.g. ball, brick, envelope and button) and asked to tell the examiner about each one.

Although the test is lengthy, the design allows plenty of warm-up time and demonstrates items in each section. This is particularly important for language-disordered children who often find a sudden change in task difficult to cope with. This assessment really does look at how well children manipulate language. Apart from very obvious differences between auditory and visual skills, in which the visual is nearly always superior, the clinician can begin to judge from the responses what language is available to the child. For example, in the auditory association subtest some children may be slow but accurate responders (Lees, 1989). There is also evidence that a small subgroup of language-impaired children have specific problems with the visual reception subtest (Urwin, Cook and Kelly, 1988). Internal reasoning is certainly required when children manipulate concepts. Some language-impaired children comment on their responses or reason out loud; they should not be penalised for doing so. It may give a good indication of the strategies they are using to succeed with complex language tasks.

The subtests may be used separately and selectively. An examiner's certificate is required in order to administer the test.

Clinical Evaluation of Language Functions (CELF)

The CELF assessment (Semel and Wiig, 1987) may well surpass the ITPA in time. It is also fairly lengthy and contains similar association and definition type tasks. It is suitable for the age range 6–18 years, but is divided further into two age groups: 5–7 years and 8–18 years. Both contain 11 subtests. Clear instructions are given for obtaining the baseline and ceiling scores which mark the individual child's starting and end point on each subtest. Tests of receptive language include the following.

Linguistic concepts

The child is required to point to an appropriately coloured line on a card after verbal instructions are given. For example, 'Before you point to a blue line, point to a red line'. There are 20 items in this section.

Sentence structure

The child has to point to the correct picture from a choice of four after verbal instructions are given. For example, 'The girl is not climbing' or 'The girl is wearing a rain coat even though she doesn't need it'. This section contains 26 items.

Oral directions

A series of circles, squares and triangles are provided and commands of increasing complexity are given which the child must carry out. These include spatial relationships and understanding sequences. There are 22 items. For the 5–7 year range an example would be, 'Point to the first big black triangle'. The same material is used for the 8–18 year age group, but the commands are more complex, for example, 'Point to the small circle, point to the biggest triangle, point to the small black square. Go!'.

Word classes

The child has to listen to four items and verbally respond with the pair which is contained within the group of four. For example, within the group 'tiger, lion, tree, baby' the pair would be 'tiger, lion'. There are 27 items in this subtest leading up to the hardest item which is 'below, away, mile, distant' to which 'away, distant' is the correct response.

Semantic relationships

The child points to two possible correct answers from a choice of four after a verbal question. For example, 'Birds are faster than . . . . . ?'. Possible answers include 'turtles, rockets, kites, planes'. There are 28 items.

Tests of expressive language include the following.

Word structure

This is a subtest which looks at plurals, personal possessives and possessive pronouns. The child looks at a picture and completes the phrase or sentence given verbally. For example, 'Here is one dog. Here are two . . . . . .'. The correct response is 'dogs'. There are 36 items altogether.

Formulated sentences

The child is given a word to put into a verbal sentence (14 items of this type). There are a further six items where the child is given two words to put into one verbal sentence. Picture material is included as an additional cue although this is not always very helpful, particularly in the harder items for the 8–18 year age group.

Recalling sentences

The child repeats a given sentence of which there are 26. The score allows for four or more errors in the repetition: score 3 for no errors, 2 for one error, 1 for two errors and 0 for four or more errors.

Sentence assembly

The child is provided with written labels and verbal instructions to construct sentences. There are 22 items and more than one correct response is possible. For example, from the labels 'saw', 'the dog', 'the woman', the child must construct two sentences: 'the woman saw the dog' and 'the dog saw the woman'.

Additional tests include the following.

Listening to paragraphs

There are two age groups of 5–9;11 years and 10 years and over. In the younger age group a simple three-line paragraph is read aloud by the examiner followed by three questions. The child responds verbally. For older children the paragraphs have nine lines and four questions are asked.

Word associations

This is a timed test. The child is allowed 60 seconds in which to name, for example, as many animals as he or she can think of or as many ways to get from one place to another.

Both the receptive and expressive language subtotals can be converted to standard scores. This allows the examiner to determine the significance of each value separately, as well as the significance of the difference between receptive and expressive abilities. Age-equivalent scores are also available. This test which has been used in some research studies (Cooper and Flowers, 1987) has been found to be useful with teenagers who are often a difficult age group for formal language testing. On the whole, the material is well produced and interesting, although some of the vocabulary is culturally exclusive (the test is from the USA).

The Aston Index: A screening procedure for written language difficulties

The Aston Index (Newton and Thompson, 1976) is included here because it is a thorough and well-researched screening test which sets out to analyse skills that are prerequisite to reading, and therefore closely related to verbal language learning. The index is designed for the age range 5–10 years and is divided into two sections: 'general underlying abilities' and 'performance items'. The first section includes a vocabulary test, a draw-a-man test, matrices, a reading test and a graded spelling test. The second section includes some sequential memory tests and sound discrimination and sound-blending tasks. The scores from the two sections are plotted on two profiles and from this the child's various strengths and weaknesses can be ascertained, both individually and in relation to the peer group. The authors argue that it is possible to identify an 'at risk' profile. They claim that the best predictors of later reading difficulty are the auditory sequential memory and sound-blending subtests. The Aston Index is most useful for a child who has a rather diffuse, high level, language problem with reported general learning and reading difficulties in school. Teachers may be fairly familiar with the test which provides a common ground when discussing intervention strategies (see Chapter 6).

Two questions summarise the use of formal tests:

1. Does the test suit the child?
2. Will it tell you what you want to know?

This will depend *what* it is you do want to know. For those wishing to compare the child with the peer group, it will be necessary to refer to how the test was standardised. The child's strengths and weaknesses may be determined, in part, by looking at the profile that is obtained or by looking in greater detail at individual responses. However, attempting to interpret what the score means in terms of functional language may well be stretching the test to its limits. The information obtained is only about the limited behaviour that has been sampled. In trying to relate this to a treatment programme, a wider range of observations is usually required.

The test results should allow the identification of areas to be focused on as a possible starting point for further analysis of assessment and within the therapy situation. This leads on to the need to use non-standardised assessments, which may follow a formal procedure and developmental guidelines, but which are less rigid in their interpretation. These will tend to sample particular areas of a skill more thoroughly. Therefore, areas appropriate for treatment emerge as a more natural progression of the assessment process. In fact, some of these procedures include a suggested language programme.

Derbyshire Language Scheme (DLS)

It is difficult to know what to say about the Derbyshire Screening Test and the Derbyshire Detailed Test of Comprehension (Knowles and Masidlover, 1982) that has not already been said in numerous workshops and teaching groups across the country. Although originally intended for use with children with severe learning difficulties, they have been used successfully in a variety of settings including language units. The schemes are well researched and have a wide appeal. However, initially at least, they are not easy to administer; the examiner needs to become quite skilled and practised at the assessment in order to be as relaxed and informal as possible. This is necessary in order to present the large number of items and score them accurately. They give clear indications as to areas of difficulty which translate directly to future treatment ideas and techniques. Key points include:

1. The test includes a variety of natural play situations which have a hidden formal procedure. This allows the examiner to focus on how many information-carrying words the child needs to understand in order to carry out a command in a particular context. For example, if the clinician provided a teddy and a sponge and said 'wash teddy', the child does not need to understand the words but only the situation. If the clinician then added a doll to the group of objects and repeated the instruction 'wash teddy', then the child would have to make a choice. A correct response would require understanding at a one-word level (i.e. that the child had understood the word 'doll' as opposed to 'teddy'). Furthermore, if a doll and a comb were added to the group of objects, the child would need to understand both 'wash' and 'teddy' in order to correctly carry out the command. This is a two-word level of understanding.
2. The emphasis is on what the child can do, so every effort is made to find the level at which the child succeeds.
3. The comprehension of grammar and vocabulary are assessed in a developmental sequence with plenty of functional examples. As a result of this 'everyday' approach to language, it is quite a straightforward exercise to develop treatment programmes for home and school from the information obtained.
4. Similarly the expression section entails a fairly easy no-nonsense grammatical analysis for those who do not feel particularly competent to carry out vast linguistic analyses.

The Derbyshire Language Scheme has a wealth of good ideas which translate to many, but not every, clinical setting. Since it is essentially a very highly structured language stimulation procedure, it is not useful for language-disordered children with very poor attention. This particular group of non-starters initially needs a rather different approach.

The Wolfson Assessment (Cooper, Moodley and Reynell, 1978)

This developmental screening procedure has been surpassed by the Derbyshire in some respects, but does include a wide range of subtests which can entail minimal language input. It includes an analysis of the child's attention level which is very important for the non-starters mentioned above. For ease of reference it will be included here. It has been further revised by Reynell (1980) and this is a summary of her descriptive framework.

Attention levels (Reynell, 1980)

Attention control	*Language as a directive function*
Level 1: 0–1 year Can pay fleeting attention but any new event will distract	Language interferes with attention
Level 2: 1–2 years Will attend to own choice of activity, but will not tolerate intervention, particularly verbal. Attention is single channelled	Language interferes with attention Must ignore other stimuli in order to concentrate on chosen activity
Level 3: 2–3 years Still single channelled Will attend to adults choice of activity, but still difficult to control	Child must stop playing to attend to adult's Must listen and then shift attention back to activity with adult help
Level 4: 3–4 years Single channelled, but more easily controlled	Adult verbalisation of task helps. Can shift attention between task and adult
Level 5: 4–5 years Integrated attention for short spell Attention span still short	Normal school entrant Child listens to instructions without interrupting activity to look at speaker Child externalises language
Level 6: 5–6 years Integrated attention is well controlled and sustained	Mature school entrant Child internalises language

Some of the subtests involving less language include: visual memory, matching, sorting, brick building and copying tasks. The following are some examples.

Visual memory

The clinician picks up one, two or even three objects from an array of eight to ten objects (which is made up of four to five pairs of objects like brush and comb, sock and shoe). These objects are then hidden from view, and then, by verbal command, key word, gesture or sign (whatever is appropriate to the child concerned), the child is instructed to find the same object.

Matching

The child is required to match a toy to a picture, which are initially identical, but gradually become less so. Secondly, the child is required to match a gesture to a picture, e.g. eating or sleeping.

Sorting

The child is required to sort items like spoons, bricks, cars etc. The clinician notes the child's ability to cope with large numbers, whether they lose concentration and/or continue to make similar errors.

Brick building and construction

The child is required to build a variety of models which are graded for difficulty. The models have names like 'wall' (a horizontal line of three bricks), 'bridge' (three bricks arranged so that one is balanced on the other two over a space). These increase in difficulty up to a set of 10 brick steps. The child may be left with the model, and the clinician may determine if the child is helped by verbal guidance or by direct intervention on the adult's part (if the child can tolerate this). In the construction task, the adult builds the model but covers it up before encouraging the child to build a similar one from memory. The examiner is then able to ascertain the child's general performance level. These tasks can also be used to focus the child into a more general assessment situation before introducing more complex language tests. As with the DLS, the emphasis is on success and finding a level at which the child can achieve. Tasks can be broken down into basic elements initially, but with the intention of building or integrating more complex auditory and visual skills as the child progresses through the programme (this will be discussed further in Chapter 5).

Language Assessment, Remediation and Screening Procedure (LARSP)

LARSP (Crystal, Fletcher and Garman, 1976) is not a standardised assessment, but it does follow a developmental sequence of emerging expressive grammatical ability for children up to 4–5 years. It was the forerunner of linguistic analyses and is perhaps the most well known. It can still be criticised as a rather lengthy procedure, but those more familiar with it will have found their own way around this particular drawback.

Whilst it may be difficult to coax a language-disordered child to produce sufficient data for an analysis, and even then the child may not progress beyond stage 4 of the scale, it is fairly essential to have a systematic look at the expressive grammar of these children. They can produce the most bizarre constructions, which may be most memorable for their oddity value, but this may well be part of an underlying trend or pattern. Perhaps the most striking feature that may be noticed when studying a sample is the paucity of the grammatical forms produced and the perseverated nature of the constructions. The contrast between elicited and spontaneous language, both in amount and form, may also bear closer analysis, particularly in respect of the child's overall communicative competence. Although this technique may take a while to master, the analysis of language samples can be speeded up with a computer program (Bishop, 1984).

Observational Checklists and Developmental Scales

Receptive and Expressive Emergent Language Scale (REEL)

The major reason for including REEL (Bzoch and League, 1970) is as an example of one way of quantifying the information given by parents and caregivers. They cannot always pinpoint exactly when their child achieved a certain skill, but they do know what the child can do, how well and where he or she does it. Since they are the experts on their child's abilities, it seems sensible to listen to what they say. The REEL is suitable for very young children (1 month to 3 years) whose language development may be impaired. It scores whether certain behaviours are present, absent or emerging (which is better than pass/fail). The examiner and parent/caregiver together can identify gaps in the child's development or areas where language is developing appropriately. This joint assessment approach can have many positive effects with regard to essential parental involvement in management. Parents become more informed about how the professionals think and vice versa.

The scale gives a clear idea of developmental sequence, so that all the common misunderstandings can be cleared up at the beginning. A fairly common example of such misunderstandings is the clinical situation in which the concerned parents attend a speech therapy session with their non-speaking child, only to find that the clinician seems to be playing with him or her rather than 'getting him or her to speak'. Parents often feel that the clinic is the place for 'speech exercises' because the child can play with dolls, teddies and tea sets at home or at the toddler group. It is not uncommon for parents and other professionals to see the speech therapist as the magician who can 'make the child talk'. In such a situation, a clear outline of what needs to happen before language emerges can really help to develop a better relationship between those concerned. An opportunity to discuss the connections between play, attention, eye contact, listening and language development is important in order to put the child's developmental progress in a proper perspective alongside the commonly used remediation techniques.

Checklist of Communicative Competence

This is an extremely detailed checklist designed for newborns to 2 year olds by Gerard (1986). It deals with social development, development of play, development of the self, as well as comprehension, verbal skills and functional communication. As it is over 20 pages long, it can be used in part or whole or over a period of time, depending on particular clinical needs. It can and should be used in conjunction with parents. Although the checklist is designed to cover the first years of development, it arguably deals with skills which are still being attained well into the third year of life, so its application is probably wider than a first glance might suggest. The suggested 'age norms' are not its most important feature. Comparison with the descriptive information contained within the checklist can be more helpful. The following examples from some of the sections will help to clarify this.

Section A (simple person-oriented behaviour) and section B (response to human contact) involve the development of selective listening, looking, turn-taking and situational understanding. They also emphasise the enjoyment of the 'communication game' that the child learns to play with other human beings. 'Looking at an adult's face' and 'making noises in response to voice' are examples of these very early communication skills. These may be very poorly developed or even non-existent in language-impaired children. Section J (interaction with other children) gives examples of the young child's non-verbal interaction with peers, including pushing, hitting, cuddling, touching and taking toys, as well as imitating others, giggling and playing 'rough and tumble'. For the language-impaired child, the quality of these non-verbal behaviours can be very important when considering, e.g. whether the child would benefit from the use of a formal non-verbal communication system.

These details can be very useful when trying to assess exactly what is 'odd' about a particular child's performance. The checklist enables the therapist to go beyond the basics of comprehension and expression into other areas of development. The language problem is not just seen in isolation, but often as part of a completely disrupted system in which play, social development and pragmatic skills are all affected to varying degrees.

Informal Assessments

Developmental checklists are really just one step away from formalising clinical observations. However, such a step means that we need a clear answer to the question: What are we looking for or at in the language-disordered population?

At times the subject seems so tenuous that it is tempting to fall back on the old view that it is what the language-disordered child is not that makes him or her language disordered (see Chapter 1). In other words, the child who fails to have adequate language skills but who isn't deaf, mentally handicapped, socially disadvantaged or emotionally disturbed, must be something else. This something else is language disorder! It cannot be sufficiently emphasised how narrowing this simplistic view is for the management of language-impaired individuals (this definition by exclusion approach is considered in Chapter 1). The view has to be wider because, as discussed in Chapter 1:

1. Hearing impairment, perhaps fluctuating, may be an additional problem for the language-disordered child.
2. Children with moderate learning difficulties may also have specific problems with language development which appear to be more than just a delay consistent with their other skills.
3. Emotional and/or social development problems may be consequent or subsequent to language impairment.
4. Some language-impaired children also display mild or moderate gross or fine motor signs so that they are called 'clumsy' (Gordon and McKinlay, 1980).

We would wish to emphasise that the view of language disorder as just one syndrome does not appear to be borne out by clinical evidence (see Chapters 1 and 3). We support a multifactorial view of the aetiology of language disorders, in which there are a range of subtypes, dependent on several paths of delayed and deviant language development. This, in turn, influences our suggestions for informal assessment of language-impaired children.

The following section is a description (with examples) of a personal view of the informal assessment of any language-disordered child. The examples are not particularly 'novel', but essentially practical.

General considerations including behaviour

There seems to be no key text which deals with the effect a severe communication disorder in one child has on family dynamics, parental control and general child behaviour, including siblings. Clezy (1978) deals with aspects of this problem, but there appear to be few others. At initial presentation the language-disordered child may appear as simply 'horrible'. There may be a story of constant temper tantrums, lack of social graces or appropriate manners, aggression towards parents, siblings and others, or the child may generally act below his or her age level. However, this is not always the picture and some may be very quiet and almost entirely non-verbal, as well as very anxious and sometimes even appearing withdrawn. Almost all of them will not tolerate the interference and guidance of an adult in any activity, although a few present more positively and seem eager to have a go at anything right from initial contact. Parents often say how they feel helpless and unable to deal with the child; they find themselves making endless compromises in their management of the child within the family, including ignoring bad behaviours, trying to protect the child and denying anything is wrong or trying desperately to coach him or her into speech and language to prove he or she is not stupid. Therefore, at the initial interview it is interesting to hear about the child's attempts to communicate within the home environment. Some real life examples include the following stories:

1. A 4-year-old child who walked across the table to get the ketchup bottle, being unable to ask.
2. A 3;6-year-old child who constantly hit her parents in the chest when requesting or initiating 'converation'.
3. A 4-year-old child who disappeared completely under the mother's clothing when conversation was directed at him.

Coping with the problem of having a language-disordered child is a serious need for parents, and should not be treated lightly by professionals. Ways of dealing with a stressful day may include splashing in the bath or screaming in the toilet, but parents should be able to discuss specific management issues with experienced individuals. A psychologist may be the best person to help to develop a programme, although general ideas can also be shared between parents within a support group. For these reasons a thorough description of any behavioural elements of the problem is essential right from the first assessment. It leads on to the problems being tackled in partnership (see Chapter 4 for management of these issues).

Attention control

Poor attention control is very common in language-disordered children, and it needs to be described accurately before any language work can begin. Poor attention control may be overt or covert. A highly distractible child is fairly obvious; less obvious is the child who has created a bland, uninterested look but who appears to be thinking about what you said until you notice the glazed expression. Many clinicians probably already find the levels of attention described earlier useful (Reynell, 1980).

It is important to create an assessment environment in which the child can succeed and one of the most important aspects of this will be to consider the attention level you expect the child to operate at. Most young, language-disordered children operate at levels 1 and 2 and a few will present for initial assessment at level 3. An overall view of the general level of attention may be clearly seen, e.g. highly distractible or attending to a choice of activities. The next important consideration is the way in which the child copes with any language that is introduced. A range of responses may include:

1. Avoidance of eye contact – literally shutting the speaker out.
2. Looking fixedly at the speaker but clearly attending elsewhere – this still shuts the speaker out, but is rather more subtle.
3. Chattering constantly and using 'empty' speech – the child simply does not allow the adult to get a word in and so puts off the need to comprehend the task in hand.
4. Running away – the child distances him- or herself from the adult and the task.
5. Beginning to throw the toys previously played with, at least demonstrating that the task is too difficult. The child may be frustrated, fed up, non-comprehending, naughty or a combination of these.
6. Picking up several things at once – the child appears to know that a response is required, but this may indicate non-comprehension and panic.
7. Generally withdrawn – the child appears reluctant to respond and also to 'fail'.

The usual form of play

It is also important to describe how the child behaves when playing in his or her preferred manner, without interference. It is not uncommon to observe the child choosing the same abstract/constructional toy each time, e.g. choosing the simple form board or bricks. Language-impaired children often confine themselves to playing with the familiar. This may be because they have a poorly defined internal framework of reference within which to develop new routines and ideas. Many factors may be involved in this tendency, including poorly developed symbolic, conceptual and cognitive skills (Griffiths, 1969; Leonard, 1979; Johnston and Ramstad, 1983). Thus the child may perform the same stereotyped action carried out repeatedly with a few toys (e.g. lines several things up, pushes things backwards and forwards) demonstrating an inability to develop a sequence of actions from the basic ability to manipulate the objects.

The assessment of play is discussed later in this chapter. In summary, while explorative and manipulative play may vary, symbolic play is almost always poor in language-disordered children (Cooper, Moodley and Reynell, 1978; Udwin and Yule, 1983). The exception to this is the child with excellent comprehension skills but little or no expressive language and at least level 3 attention. He or she may be observed acting out fairly complex play sequences with miniature toys, and may accompany this with intonation patterns, often to the exclusion of any other type of play. It may be thought that play has become the vehicle of expression and often the behaviour dwindles as expressive language improves.

Problem solving

It is important to see if the child can solve any of the problems present in the environment, e.g. using a pile of boxes to allow him or her to reach the door handle of the room where the toys are kept. Other related examples would be the spontaneous use of gestures and 'props' to aid communication, e.g. finding a pair of glasses to indicate that the person intended in the unidentified utterance was a grandparent. Such activities require the child to develop an idea, hold it in memory and then to adapt and modify it according to the situation.

Improving performance – techniques and strategies

Anything that seems to help the child to function better should be considered; this could include:

1. A quiet environment in which distractions are minimal.
2. Using gesture or sign system, facial expression and eye glides as additional visual cues.
3. Using key words or just single words like 'listen' and 'look' to cue the child into a demonstration.
4. Physically turning the child's face towards the adult (or the child turning the adult's face to her- or himself).
5. Making the immediate rewards of successful communication obvious with praise and facial expression, as the child is usually highly bound to the present situation.
6. The increased motivation which comes from finishing even a simple task; initially activities need to be very short and visually rewarding.

Once the child completes tasks and finds success rewarding, he or she will respond more appropriately to future praise and censure. This has a powerful 'knock on' effect in other environments. Invariably, in our experience, the child wants to please the adult. This usually has the effect of making her or him less difficult to manage in various environments, both home, clinic and toddler group. Improved cooperation makes language problems easier to assess and manage.

Most children will perform one or two tasks at the initial assessment, although it may be necessary to use all of the above techniques to facilitate this. Here is an example of such a situation:

> *Case 6* (see also Chapter 4)
> A girl aged 3;3 years was thought to have normal hearing. At the initial assessment there was an increase in fluent but empty speech, which gradually became more bizarre, when she was required to listen to anything. This language included utterances like: 'Oh what's your name, Oh look over there, Oh what's the time, How much is that doggy in the window', and much more.
>
> Her attention was at level 1 at best and it was difficult for her to achieve anything. It took many attempts before she could stop talking and sit still momentarily. Further progress was made by physically turning her head to look at the adult and then taking her hand to help her put a brick into a posting box, all using minimal language but a lot of praise and encouragement. By this method the assessment session revealed some information about the child's needs (to improve attention as a precursor to further assessment of verbal comprehension), as well as demonstrating to the child, parent and therapist that it was possible for the child to succeed at a simple task.

Physical appearance, gait and facial features

There could already be clues about this from the case history. The parents may have reported slow motor development, poor coordination, messy eating, variability of performance which is difficult to quantify, persistent dribbling or poor organisational skills. Any of these may be demonstrated during the assessment, while the child is playing or having a drink, for example; however, this could be the first time that any of this information has been given careful consideration, perhaps highlighting the need for a further medical examination, and will be discussed in detail in Chapter 3.

Assessment Ideas: Tasks and Materials

The clinician may already have, or wish to make, a portable informal assessment that will cope with just about anything. Equally he or she may prefer to take equipment from one shelf or nursery cupboard according to age or experience of the child, or even follow the child's lead or choice (although this is not feasible if the child is highly distractible). Whatever the eventual method or choice of materials, activities should be constructed which can assess particular aspects of behaviour as accurately as possible. For example take a verbal comprehension task which requires the child to select an object on request from a range of five. If the child fails the task the following questions should be asked:

1. Was the child attending?
2. Was the child attending for long enough?
3. Was the child distracted by the choice offered?
4. Was the child distracted by the language used?
5. Was this due to the content of the phrase?
6. Was it the question form that was not understood?

It would be uncertain which one factor or combination of factors was operating, if the activity was carried out in isolation. The task initially appeared simple enough, but in fact we can see that it is too complex a starting point.

For the distractible child, it is necessary first to establish the best way of gaining the child's attention. Then it is possible to increase gradually the number of object choices presented and finally add the language (either 'Show me .....' or 'Where's the ....' and see which one works best). Manipulating these variables ensures a pattern of success so that, at the first point of failure, a fairly accurate clinical judgement can be made, based on previous observations. Begin with a variety of performance tasks, rather than plunging straight into an assessment of verbal comprehension. This will allow for greater flexibility on the part of the adult to use demonstration, cues and gestures and, in this way, establish a relationship with the child.

A number of visual tasks which vary in complexity can then be introduced. Initially, they can be used to enable the child to focus his or her attention without language and achieve some success, as well as to establish a relationship with the examiner and to demonstrate what the child *can* do. More complex visual material can also be used to work with and establish integrated attention and pre-reading skills. When selecting materials, it is also useful to consider other variables, such as manual dexterity, physical movement and hand–eye coordination. In addition some activities could include a visual sequencing or memory component. For screening purposes a portable assessment need only include three activities at a basic, middle and higher level.

Visual/visuomotor activities

Age level	Material	Questions
Preschool	Posting box/van/men in boat	How quickly does the child learn or cooperate?
3–7+ years	Floorshapes: large geometric shapes scattered on floor, child copies adult route from two or more shapes	Can child hold a sequence in memory while moving?
	Form boards and puzzles	Are abstract ones or objects/people preferred?
3–5 years	Construction tasks using bricks (trains, houses)	Can child copy designs? Can child construct one from memory?
5–9 years	Using Lego (car, plane, rocket, robot)	What does the child build spontaneously?
3–6 years	Visual memory for objects (5–10 pairs of objects), e.g. using animal shapes	Can the child remember the hidden object?
5–8 years	Smaller objects and more in array, adult hides two to three	Can the child remember a sequence?
	Visual memory for pictures using cards differing only slightly	Does the child match on one criterion only?
	Spot the differences in complex pictures	Can the child scan effectively from one to another?

Conceptual development: assessment activities

Initially these tasks involve simple matching and sorting skills, but, as they become more complex, they gradually require more than just visual ability. With each subsection, the language used also becomes more complex. They are arranged here to reflect a developmental progression.

Activities	*Comments*
1. Sorting	
(a) objects: cars, beads, shapes	Is the attention level affected by the number of things being sorted?
(b) pictures: hats, clocks, shoes	Does the child need fairly constant attention — verbal or non-verbal?
2. Classification	Picture cards can be useful here. The
(a) food, transport, clothes, musical instruments	language component can be altered, added to or reduced as necessary
(b) domestic objects, rooms (bathroom, kitchen)	It should be possible to adapt lotto games by placing a box by each board so that the child sorts the cards into each box
(c) animals	
(d) land, sea, sky (associated objects, people, animals etc.)	Look to see if the child has to hunt for the items in the 'scene' or if he or she classifies according to previous knowledge
(e) pairs, find a pair of things that go together (glove/hand, baby/cot)	Does the child need adult direction? Can the child manage more than one card at a time?
3. Size	
(a) objects: big/little	Any play material may be used
(b) pictures: shark/goldfish, jumbo jet/glider	At an easier stage provide boxes for sorting little and big things Do gestures help the child?
4. Time	
(a) sequence card stories	Plenty of material is available. However, it can be a good idea to photograph the child doing things over time
(b) more abstract: seasons, days of the week, time in the day	Can they recall them? What happens during the day? Are props or picture cues needed to aid sequencing abilities (pyjamas, food, coat, book)?
5. Place: prepositions	
(a) obstacle course	For young children two-dimensional material is hard to interpret. Objects are better. If using photos they must be clear
(b) finding objects or pictures	Children need real experience of being in, on, under, in front of, behind each other
6. Number	
(a) more, same using cars, bricks or juice	It is worth checking this concept as even older children may be failing at a basic level
(b) add one, take one away and number symbols	Dominoes and board games can be adapted for this

Symbolic development: assessment activities

In general, language-disordered children are not adept at manipulating symbols. Trying to find the level at which this breakdown occurs requires a step-wise approach. Some basic tasks should be included as well as the more complex material, so that a hierarchy is built up that allows the whole to be assessed in small logical steps. When selecting material, consider the mode of presentation (i.e. verbal or gestural). Initially a demonstration, 'key words' or signs/gestures may be all the child can tolerate when comprehension and attention are also very poor.

Activity	Comment
1. Preschool children	
(a) Matching life-sized objects to large doll play material (cup, spoon, brush, sock, toothbrush)	These may seem less appropriate for a portable assessment but they can be used in later play sessions
(b) Matching large doll to dolls house sized play material (cup, spoon, doll, blanket, dress, trousers)	These early stages can often help the distractible child focus in on the task and then cope with later material
	The child may not need to label items but demonstrate function of object on self or doll
(c) Matching dolls house sized items to very similar pictures (bed, chair, bath, cup)	
(d) Matching small objects to less similar pictures (toy house to photo of house, racing car to photo of taxi)	
(e) Matching gesture to picture (eating, sleeping, drinking, driving)	Once attending the language-impaired child is usually adept at interpreting gesture
2. For school age children (up to 10 years old) The visual reception subtest of the ITPA	This subtest can give information about the child's ability to match symbols at quite a complex level

Symbolic play

Play may be exploratory, physical, constructional, imaginative and social (Jeffree, McKonky and Hewson, 1977; Garvey, Cooke and Williams, 1985). Observing the play of children in nurseries and playgrounds confirms the infinite variety of routines, experiences and emotions that children can achieve in play. Sadly, this level of sophistication is less readily available to language-disordered children (Udwin and Yule, 1983). In general, language-disordered children do not appear to develop complex imaginative symbolic play or, if they do, it happens very slowly. Perhaps this reflects their inability to manipulate and sequence ideas and events (Cooper, Moodley and Reynell, 1978). It is preferable to assess play at home or in a nursery setting, where familiar toys are available. This way the clinician can see what the child selects. For the language-disordered child, experience suggests that this is usually cars, puzzles, lego or nothing at all.

However, it is not always possible to carry out long assessments in the home or nursery (particularly when speech therapy resources are scarce). It may be necessary to set up play situations in order to observe and record the child's behaviour. In order to do this a variety of play items will be required. Here are some suggestions which have proved useful in practice:

1. For large doll play: teddy, doll or similar, tea set, washing and washing up items, bed and bedclothes.
2. For small doll play: a selection of dolls house furniture and small people, a small set of animals and tractor, or small people within a playground scene or garage.
3. For role-playing or dressing up: a variety of hats, bags, gloves, cloaks, jackets etc.

A checklist can be useful for focusing observations. Gerard (1986) includes a detailed section on play but it may be too lengthy for some clinical situations. A more concise format, including descriptions of child interaction and play behaviour is outlined below.

Levels of child interaction

Example	Comment
1. Approximately 9–18 months: The child does not allow the play routine to be altered If this is attempted it may be ignored, or the child may become angry or move away For example, an adult builds a tower of blocks for the baby to knock over. After 20 or so turns, the adult attempts to change the shape of the tower to stairs. The baby becomes agitated and pushes the adult's hand away	The language-disordered child presenting at 3 years can be typically at this stage of development Characteristically, play routines are brief and cannot be altered or added to. The child will not tolerate any interference

Example	*Comment*
2. Approximately 18–24 months: The child allows an adult or peer to play alongside, but does not adapt to play with another Again, if the adult tries to alter the routine the toddler may reject this in various ways (snatching the item away, throwing it, pushing adult aside)	Language-disordered children have a tendency for solitary play. They may be aware of others and take toy items from them but rarely cooperate with peers
3. Approximately 2–3 years: The child begins to seek adult involvement The child can produce short play routines (like making tea, putting dolly to bed), but often refers to the adult model to sustain and evolve play	When language-disordered children accept adult guidance, verbal or non-verbal, the parents/therapist can begin to teach and model play sequences
4. Approximately 3–4 years: The child enjoys interaction with other children for short periods The child can also sustain play alone without an adult to facilitate this In children developing language normally a verbal commentary accompanies this	There are a few young language-disordered children who come for assessment at this level. Their symbolic play is complex and solitary, verbal comprehension is within normal limits or above average but expressive language is usually non-existent (Urwin, Cook and Kelly, 1988)
5. Approximately 4–5 years and above: The child enjoys cooperative games for short periods (dressing up, Wendy house play, large constructional play) The child really needs language as a mediator at this stage A typical 4 year old will usually argue and interrupt By 5 years cooperative play is well sustained. The child understands the rules and the concepts of sharing and turn-taking	Preschool language-disordered children rarely cooperate at this level of play. Physical contact is still the usual mediator

Types of play behaviour

(Child presented with symbolic play toys like cup, comb, spoon, doll, teapot etc.)

Example	*Comment*
1. Under 12 months: Inappropriate or nil response The child throws the toys or piles them up. There may be a tendency to fiddle mechanically with the toys The child may walk away and ignore the toys	This type of response is often a result of non-comprehension of the toy's potential. It is typical of the language-disordered child with poor attention
2. Over 12 months: Showing understanding by use The child may stir the cup with the spoon, comb their own or the doll's hair. The actions do not constitute a sequence of ideas but rather are isolated events	Older language-disordered children (over 3 years) often group items together (place the doll on a chair, chair by table). This is sometimes described as symbolic play but is in fact an earlier stage
3. Approximately 18–24 months: The child develops short play sequences These are usually domestic and similar in nature (pouring out the tea, stirring it, giving doll a drink)	Language-disordered children can be observed using the items but need direct help to sequence ideas and actions
4. Approximately 2–3 years: The child plays in short, complex and dynamic sequences The child enjoys imitating other children and adults and repeating favourite routines over and over again	Language-disordered children with good attention control enjoy participating in play sequences with an adult
5. Over 3 years: The child makes up novel sequences and personalised routines Imaginative symbolic play is dynamic and it does not depend on 'props' or a particular context (Garvey, 1982) For example, the 2;6-year-old son of one of the authors who said he had a 'tiny yellow frog on his hand'. It lived in his bedroom and jumped all over the bed	Language-disordered children may become adept at imitating and enjoying complex play routines, appearing very competent. However, they may be unable to evolve their own sequences. They may carry out well-known, learned sequences particularly if the 'props' and context are the same (i.e. the clinic room)

Verbal comprehension

Various structures are possible for this section, but the model advocated by the Derbyshire Language Scheme (Knowles and Masidlover, 1982) is a particularly popular one. The scheme was discussed earlier in the chapter. In outline, the model enables practised users of the scheme to assess verbal comprehension and expressive language skills at various levels of complexity via structured play situations. If you are unfamiliar with the scheme, making the assessment seem natural and extracting all the relevant information can be daunting. It takes time to master the necessary skills. It is not recommended that a clinician tries to put it into operation without attending a course. However, this does not mean that therapists cannot adopt the general principles of the model and perhaps include similar ideas within their own informal assessment. The areas to focus on can include the following.

Information carrying words

How much information can the child process? To begin with, single word commands are called key words. When combined within commands the number of information carrying words present will vary depending on the situational clues provided.

1. To assess comprehension of key words the following can be used: objects, pictures of objects, miniature toys, actions, pictures of actions, parts of body (own and dolls)
2. Relating two bits of information:
   Put <u>dolly</u> in <u>bed</u>
   Where's the <u>teddy's</u> <u>nose</u>
   Wash dolly
   Who's sitting on the bed
   Where's the dog walking
   Wash dolly's hands
   Which one do you drink from
3. Relating three bits of information (prepositions, relative size):
   Put <u>baby</u> <u>under</u> the <u>box</u>
   <u>Wash</u> <u>teddy's</u> <u>face</u> (from a choice of doll, teddy, comb and sponge)
   Put the dolly under the table
   Make baby dance on the chair
   Give the little spoon to dolly
   Put the spoon in teddy's cup
   Where's the man climbing the ladder
4. Relating four bits of information:
   Make daddy sit down under the table
   Put the baby under the big bed

Comprehension of syntax

This can be examined at both sentence and word level. Once again, both play and picture material could be used to assess them. Ten categories of sentence structure are suggested:

1. Verb phrase: the boy is eating an ice cream.
2. Preposition phrase: the girl is between her mum and dad.
3. Wh questions: Who is that?
4. Modifiers: the dog has a big blue ball.
5. Negatives: the girl is not walking.
6. Passives: the boy is being chased by the bull.
7. Infinitives: the boy wanted to swim across the pool.
8. Relative clauses: the cat that is black is eating some fish.
9. Subordinate clauses: the baby is crying because she wants some dinner.
10. Indirect request: Shouldn't you take your coat off?

Six categories of word level comprehension are suggested:

1. Plurals (regular and irregular): book/books, man/men, sheep/sheep.
3. Possession: Matthew's, Mum's
3. Past tense (regular and irregular): jump/jumped, write/wrote, get/got.
4. Personal pronouns: her, hjm.
5. Possessive pronouns: his, hers.
6. Demonstratives: that, those, these.

Here are some examples of the types of sentences which could be used for Wh questions:

> Who can't get the apples?
> Why can't he reach it?
> Who's eaten her dinner?
> Who isn't eating?
> Who is going to bed?
> Where's the man standing next to the car?

Vocabulary

The areas of vocabulary the child should be familiar with should include vocabulary from the home situation as well as from other familiar environments. Once again these are just suggestions which could be assessed using play and picture material in a variety of ways:

Home environment
    Family names.
    Common everyday activities: meals, bath time etc.

Specific family items including pets if relevant.

General household items including clothes and furniture.

Other familiar environments

Activities that relate directly to the child: running, sliding, falling, rolling, sleeping etc.

Places the child is familiar with: park, playground, shop.

Items in those places: swing, slide, trolley, basket.

Favourite television programmes and their characters: Thomas the Tank Engine and Postman Pat are frequently admired by young language-disordered children.

The vocabulary of basic concepts

Direction and position: up, on, in, open, close.

Size: big, small, fat, thin.

Emotions: happy, sad, poorly.

Other attributes: cold, hot, shiny, smooth, hard.

Time: old, new, today, yesterday, first, next.

Number: the numbers 1 to 10, more, less, same.

Colour: the primary colours and pink, brown, black and white.

Shape: circle, round, square, triangle, star.

The wider environment

Two different large topic areas could be chosen like the seaside, town, zoo or space. A range of items such as transport, animals and other living things, people doing different jobs or wearing different clothes, and more unusual things like weather, could be provided in picture form. The clinician is interested to see if the child can classify and cross-reference his or her knowledge when selecting which items belong in which environment. It is also interesting to see if the child is able to give further examples from his or her experience (e.g. 'We go on a bus', 'I saw Star Wars', 'It bit me').

Expressive skills

This section aims to look at more than just verbal skills as a measure of expressive ability in language-disordered children. Severely reduced verbal output may well be an obvious feature, or conversely the child could be a fluent speaker whose utterances are characterised by bizarre and inappropriate content which appear tangential in nature (this is not easy to assess – see Adams and Bishop, 1989; Bishop and Adams, 1989). However, it is important to observe the child's behaviour and evaluate what he or she does in response to difficulties with sentence formulation. A range of coping strategies may emerge. These may be positive (uses gestures and cues to aid communication), negative (bites those who fail to understand) or there may be no strategies at all (child loses interest in communication and walks away). The types of strategies a child employs will be important when considering treatment programmes aimed at increasing effective communication (see Chapter 4). Here are some of the factors which need to be considered in the assessment of a child's expressive skills.

Situational aspects

It is helpful to ascertain (from reports or direct observation) whether the child's expressive skills vary between one situation and another or between different people in her or his environment. For example, is the child more expressive or more withdrawn at playgroup? Does the child appear to communicate best at home? Does the child frequently resort to temper tantrums when not understood? How are these dealt with? What method(s) do the child's family/caretakers use to communicate with her or him? Do the parents and child enjoy communicating despite the difficulties?

There are no right answers to any of these questions. They are not asked with a view to building up prejudices about the child's background; their purpose is to focus observation on the communicative interchange that goes on within the family and home environment. Armed with these observations the clinician is able to be more sensitive in working with the family members towards facilitating more appropriate communication from the child. Parents may have adapted very well to the difficulties their child has with communication in the home. In such a case, it may be more relevant to attend to communication difficulties in playgroup or at nursery.

Paralinguistic aspects (the use of intonation and other vocalisations)

Not many non-verbal children are silent. Some use intonated babble or shouting and screaming to gain a hearing. Some may even cough to fill the silence. Others will use a few protowords with gesture, often using the same vocalisation in a non-specific way in many situations. Sometimes the intonation pattern that overrides the vocalisation will differ for different needs.

Use of mime, gesture and facial expression

Some language-disordered children develop their own elaborate system of gestures and signs or exaggerated facial expression and head movements with which to communicate. Some use body movement, including touching and pulling, whilst others make no use of any of these physical strategies. More passive or anxious children may appear to literally 'curl up' with head lowered, shoulders rounded and no eye contact, thus opting out of communication.

Verbal skills

Most clinicians develop a preferred method of assessing verbal language. It is important to get some idea of the range of grammatical structures, if any, that the child uses. There should be little problem in obtaining an adequate sample of verbal language from the fluent 'empty' speakers (play, pictures, role-playing, story telling or conversation may all be useful). However, children who have severe problems with word joining may produce little or nothing. In such cases, it may be necessary to elicit a sample of verbal language by using forced alternatives (e.g. 'Is this the rabbit jumping or the dog running?'), by delayed imitation or story telling. If appropriate, the parents might be asked to tape the child when he or she is more relaxed in the home environment, or they could be asked to keep a diary of utterances over a week. This may actually confirm that the child's verbal skills are confined to a few words and learned phrases.

It can be helpful to have a quick checklist of verbal language which can be used in the clinic or when visiting the home or nursery. This checklist, with examples, amalgamates several different approaches.

Expressive language checklist

	Example	*Date*

1. Single nouns and verbs:
   mummy, gone! more, no,
   allgone, there, daddy

2. Two-word phrases (N Phrase/V
   Phrase):
   no drink, daddy there,
   kick ball, my teddy,
   mummy play, gone car

3. Three-word phrases (Wh questions,
   negatives, prepositional phrases):
   Daddy wash car,
   that pretty flower,
   where Mummy gone,
   go to park now?

4. Four plus word phrases (possessives,
   plurals, past tense):
   We went to the beach
   I don't want to
   Where my mummy's hat gone?
   I got boots on

	Example	*Date*

5. Complex phrases (coordination,
   subordination, tagged and
   comparative clauses):
   Mummy and me went to the shops
   and I got sweets and I felled over.
   It's bigger than that!
   You bettern't do that.

6. Complex phrases (passive, complex
   verb phrase complement):
   I got kicked.
   It was when you had just been born,
   Katie.
   also use of: must, may,
   should, all both, much, many

However, syntax is not the only variable. It is also important to assess the child's range of expressive vocabulary. Language-disordered children may have difficulty in learning, storing and retrieving vocabulary (Haynes, 1982). Typically this is manifest as a paucity in the content of expressive language. Children may continue to use the wrong words (perseveration) or, in failing to produce the target words, produce phonemic or semantic errors instead (paraphasias). A look at expressive vocabulary could be carried out using the same material recommended for vocabulary in the comprehension section. Once again a range of techniques might be required to elicit an adequate sample of this including pretend play, role-playing and story telling.

Use of language

It has recently become rather popular to consider the way in which children use language to communicate: their pragmatic skills. Whilst it may be an overgeneralisation, the majority of language-impaired children are thought to have poor pragmatic skills, which is perhaps an obvious consequence of never having been very good at using this medium. Others have a pragmatic disorder and, over the last 10 years, various attempts have been made to define this (Gallagher and Prutting, 1983; McTear, 1985; Shielfelbusch and Pikar, 1986; Adams and Bishop, 1989; Bishop and Adams, 1989). Three main areas of pragmatic ability have been identified which interact depending on the child's context.

1. Communicative intent: both the range and the form of these intents should be considered. The range includes such intents as to request, comment, respond, protest, reject, greet, gain attention or regulate conversation. The form might be either verbal or non-verbal from

gesture, one word, or many words. The normally developing child should demonstrate various types and forms of intent at all stages.

2. Organisation of discourse: this would include turn-taking, topic initiation and maintenance, topic breakdown and repair and termination of discourse strategies.

3. Presupposition: this includes sharing information and understanding communication from the perspective of the listener. The child needs to be aware of different social contexts, settings and communication channels.

Dore (1975) identified six types of behaviour that he termed speech acts. These were said to account for all the intended messages used by a fluent speaker at the multiword stage of development. These behaviours are presented here in the form of a checklist, with examples, which could be used as a framework within which to evaluate the language-impaired child's pragmatic abilities.

Checklist of pragmatic abilities

1. Range of communicative intents:
    (a) Requesting information: Where's Mum?
    (b) Requesting action: Don't do that!
    (c) Responding to requests: Alright, here's one.
    (d) Stating or commenting: This is my car. I don't like dogs.
    (e) Regulating conversation: Yes, I see. Hello. Guess what?
    (f) Other performatives including teasing, warning or conveying humour: Watch out!
2. Organisation of discourse:
    (a) Turn-taking: when to change the subject and interrupt as well as how to use questions, eye gaze or facial expression to complete a clause.
    (b) Attention seeking and directing devices: non-verbal including touch, gesture and facial expression as well as verbal requests and regulators like: Yes, but .... or Well, I .....
    (c) Initiation: in the young child these will be directed to the self: I got juice.
    (d) Reinitiation: a whole or part repetition of the phrase or a rephrase: May I have it now ..... may I have it!
    (e) Responding: there might be no response, inappropriate response, appropriate response, minimal response or a response with additional information.
    (f) Initiation with response: this is usually a response to the previous utterance which also initiates a reply: Where are my socks? Aren't they in the draw? No!

(g) Follow-up that is evaluative or acknowledgement: used a lot by parents and therapists so the pragmatically impaired child may well pick this up: Yes, it's a man driving.

(h) Topic maintenance: non-verbally this may be a gesture, nodding, or eye gaze and verbally such things as: Yes! Really?

(i) Topic change: this is usually sensitive to context unless an abrupt change is intended for social reasons. The pragmatically impaired child rarely advances to this level of sophistication, and inappropriate topic change is usually about non-comprehension of these rules.

(j) Identification of breakdown which requests clarification: Did you mean that one?

(k) Repair: this can be self-initiated or due to another person: Get your jumper . . . . the blue one, or Get your jumper . . . . . This blue one?

(l) Termination: may be non-verbal by eye gaze, facial expression or gesture or verbal using words like: OK, bye, thanks.

3. Presupposition: shared information may be established from:

(a) An earlier sentence: My Aunty came to tea yesterday. [Did she?] Yes, and she wanted to kiss me.

(b) Previous knowledge of the person or the experience. This example only makes sense if the listener is able to supply this: We got really hot there, but it was fantastic!

(c) Knowledge of the world. This must be applied to make an example like this make sense (one parent to another at a toddler's birthday party): You must be mad!

(d) Knowledge of social contexts and personal characteristics. This different behaviour, verbal and non-verbal, may be appropriate in different situations and with specific speakers, like adult-to-child vs child-to-child interactions.

(e) Awareness of the physical context and its limitations: for example, the appropriateness of saying 'See this' over the telephone.

Such a range of information may be interesting, but how it can be used to monitor possible areas of breakdown in language-disordered children is a different question. The way in which poor pragmatic skills are differentiated from disordered ones needs to be established. Several strands of clinical research have recently looked at this (Haynes, 1986; Roux and Schneider, 1988; Adams and Bishop, 1989; Bishop and Adams, 1989). A summary of those difficulties which are considered to indicate a disorder of pragmatics is as follows:

1. The child has problems recognising communicative intent. This means that the child fails to select the relevant part of the utterance such that what is implied may be interpreted as a statement and conversational regulators are not recognised.

2. Types of verbal behaviour used by the child are limited. This means that the child may ask frequent questions but little else.
3. The child may have difficulties with the whole idea of the speaker/listener conversational flow. Thus they respond inappropriately to the adult response and initiation, question and answer due to poor insight.
4. The child is poor at turn-taking and timing of responses.
5. Slow, rigid and often bizarre concept development results in difficulties of presupposition by the child. He or she fails to make sense of the world and/or use any information in the conversational situation. Literal interpretation is a feature of this style. The child appears unable to make inferences. He or she has poor self-awareness as a group member and poor awareness of what knowledge is shared or logically entailed.

Here are some example of the kinds of pragmatic difficulties shown by language-disordered children.

Child A

Child A was 6;6 years old when this conversation with a teacher was recorded at play time:

> T: Shouldn't you get your coat?
> A: My coat?
> T: Yes, it's cold.
> A: Why? Where you going? It's play time it is. What's that, what?
> T: Get your coat please.
> A: Coatee, coatee, coatee. Stop it Jason.
> T: Listen. Get your coat. Now.
> A: OK.

Child B

Child B was 7;6 years old when he had this conversation with his teacher about an event she had not witnessed:

> T: You choose which one you would like?
> B: I want the ball. . . . I got told off I did.
> T: Did you?
> B: I threw a ball and he kicked me and I hit him and oooooh! Mrs X (head teacher) . . . . . I had to see Mrs X. It's not fair.
> T: Never mind, never mind. Let's forget that. It's all over now.
> B: Do you know Mrs X? Oh I like this ball.
> T: Don't bounce it too hard!
> B: What are we doing then?

Child C

Child C was 7 years old. He was asked by his teacher to 'Find out as much as you can about Sandra' (another child in the class).

C: Why do you wear glasses?
S: I need them to see.
C: Can't you see then?
S: Yes, but not very well.
C: My mum wears them, not my dad. Where's my dad? He's coming soon.
S: Weren't you supposed to ask me about my family. Where I live?
C: Where you live? At home.
S: Yes.
C: You have .. your are .... You have a mum? I have a mum. And my dad. Where is he?
S: Yes, but ..... [Sandra getting quite exasperated!]

Many language-disordered children just display poor pragmatic skills, rather than disordered ones, which are due to specific comprehension problems and difficulty with retrieval of syntax and vocabulary. In terms of communicative intent, the child may recognise the intent as a request or comment but have difficulty processing it. He or she may have difficulty using questions and thus requesting and initiating conversation due to poor syntactic and vocabulary development. Here is another example of a 5 year old talking to a therapist:

T: Hello, what have you got there?
D: A picture! A me!
T: Did you draw it?
D: Yeah. That mum, that dad, that Natty [sister, Natalie], that ... [unintelligible].
T: That's your dog isn't it?
D: Yeah ..... [unintelligible].
T: That's lovely. Did you do it at home?
D: Yeah.
T: Shall we put it on the wall then?
D: No ..... a take home!
T: Yes you can take it home later. If we put it here, everyone can see it. There!
D: Yeah.

In this example the child's poor pragmatic skills resulted in a difficulty of fluent exchange which appears to be due mainly to limitations of syntax and vocabulary. The child's responses were slow and limited, but not essentially inappropriate. For these children, presupposition may be underdeveloped due to slow and patchy concept development. Literal interpretation may be related to immaturity of world knowledge and a failure to generalise what he or she has. For example: a 9-year-old child shown a picture of a mother pig suckling some baby piglets responded: 'Those pigs eating the big pig'.

It may not be appropriate to include an in-depth assessment of pragmatics in the assessment of every language-disordered child, because it is such a wide area and would take some considerable time. Equally, some would argue that such an assessment would make the use of a video camera and recorder essential, which may not be available in all clinical situations. However, pragmatic skills should not just be considered as an afterthought in the assessment of the language-disordered child. They are an important consideration when trying to produce a comprehensive child-centred view of the strengths and weaknesses that contribute to the communication skills developing in any one individual. However, their complex nature and the present trends in research indicate that we still have a great deal to learn about this aspect of language development and deviancy.

From assessment to treatment

A wealth of information, test scores and observations should be available on completion of the assessment period. It is unlikely to have been accumulated in one visit or in one situation. The more complex the problem, the more time the clinician will need to spend on assessment. In some respects the assessment process is never finished, for even during the treatment phase reassessment and re-evaluation of progress is important to ensure that therapy is useful and targeted at the child's needs. However, armed with the information gained from assessment, we are now ready to discuss how this might be used in the differential diagnosis and treatment of language-disordered children.

Chapter 3
Differential Diagnosis
of Language Disorder

Summary

The complex nature of language disorder and the way this affects the developing child is of concern to a wide range of professionals. This chapter discusses how these professionals can work together in a multidisciplinary team for the effective differential diagnosis of the child's strengths and needs. This includes the value of a comprehensive case history and developmental assessment. The speech therapist's role in such a process is particularly emphasised through the use of longitudinal language assessment.

Introduction

The problem of what to call things is a common one both socially and professionally. Giving a label to a situation, condition or individual, helps you to recognise it when you see it again. Set prescriptions may exist for certain phenomena. Some may find the label helpful in demystifying the problem: if you know what it is called it cannot hurt you. For others the label only serves to create further mystery. In the field of language disorder some see the process of differential diagnosis in these terms – giving 'it' a label. Although partially justified it is not the only purpose. Differential diagnosis is about unravelling the whole situation in order to allow for appropriate forward planning for the child and family concerned.

Whilst differential diagnosis begins from first seeing a child, for those with complex language disorders it may take many years of careful evaluation of intervention and consequent progress before the condition can be named. In others the name of the syndrome is obvious from the early stages because it has a characteristic phenotype. However, a careful description of the unfolding of a disorder is ultimately more important than its name. Rarely will the name of a particular syndrome associated with language impairment result in a prescriptive treatment which will accelerate the child's language development. Treating language problems in children is much more a question of carefully detailing how the condition unfolds and the child's particular response to therapy programmes as described in Chapter 4. The major purposes of differential diagnosis are:

1. To establish a baseline for the individual child's language disorder.
2. From there to help in setting up an appropriate treatment/management plan.
3. To help the child, family and others involved to come to terms with the history and implications of the condition.
4. To help these people recognise the condition if it recurs, either in the same family or another.
5. To allow cross-child comparisons which would be helpful in clinically based research.

The way in which these tasks are carried out will depend on the clinical situation. Whilst it is possible for them all to be done separately, by different individuals, so that the child and family visit a number of professionals in different places who each make their contribution (something like a shopping expedition), this is not necessarily the most useful, productive or efficient method of establishing a differential diagnosis. Where the child and family can be seen by a multidisciplinary team which, as far as possible, operates under one roof, a more holistic picture of the child's needs is likely to emerge. However, even in places where this works well, it is rarely possible to use the same professionals to answer all the questions. More specialist knowledge may be required in some respects and greater knowledge of local resources in others. Equally, some professionals are able to work in teams and others clearly are not. Team work is not just a 'good idea' but requires a positive commitment on the part of all concerned so that all the skills available may be used for the child's best interests. We shall use the model of a multidisciplinary team for differential diagnosis and discuss its advantages and disadvantages in the light of the five purposes outlined above.

Establishing a Baseline of the Child's Language Disorder

Before deciding what to do, it is necessary to know how severe the problem is and what the child's strengths and weaknesses are. This is the process of assessment. It has a number of essential components which could be done separately but will be discussed here as if done within a team setting.

The case history

There are some clinicians who think this has gone out of fashion or that it is in some way 'nosey' to begin an interview with a case history. That probably depends on how it is done. Good case-history taking is certainly an art which can take a professional a lifetime to learn. It is obviously important at the beginning of an interview to establish a relationship with the child and family and not necessarily to begin by launching into a lot of intimidating jargon-filled questions. This is why taking a good history is much easier in a team, or at least with one other person present. It then becomes a conversation about the whole situation which is seen from many different perspectives, and not just a verbal questionnaire or some kind of clinical opinion poll. At the same time, the child has a chance to settle down and interact with family members and professionals together rather than being expected to perform straight away. Where appropriate, the child is also able to contribute to the case history with names of other siblings, ages, school attended and teachers' names etc.

Some will say that resources do not allow for the luxury of more than one person being involved in the case-history taking. This seems to be a rather short-sighted argument. Even within a busy health centre, it is possible to set up times for an initial interview which could be done with two therapists or with therapist and health visitor for example. For the family, a relaxed group situation is far less intimidating than a fierce professional behind a desk. For the professionals, a wider view of the child and family situation is provided when it is discussed by those with different experiences. Setting aside one morning or afternoon a week, or however frequently is necessary to cope with the referral rate, to which others can be invited, is probably more productive in the long term. It saves the therapist, clinical medical officer or health visitor trying to liaise with the other parties after the interview in order to fill in any other information. Secondly, the family sees that the professionals know each other and share a common concern. This is probably more reassuring than a view which suggests they never see each other and do not even know each other's names, particularly when the child has complex needs.

In a child development centre, all the professionals will be under one roof. However, this does not mean that case-history interviews and the rest of the assessment procedure are actually carried out within a multidisciplinary team. Quite often it just means that the professionals sit in their separate offices, and the child and family visit one after the other. Although it requires less 'leg work' on the part of the professional it is not really team work. Team work means being in the same place at the same time and doing it together; it means occupying the same room. Some suggest this intimidates the family and child. Experience rejects that view; a friendly, well coordinated team is no less intimidating than one over-worked and stressed professional fiercely defending a lonely office. In fact, team work should be much more supportive to family and professionals alike.

As for the case history, how should it be done? The interview should begin by establishing the parents' major concerns about the child's development. Whoever leads the case-history taking, and there are no rules about this but someone in the team may be better at it than others, should be sure to document what it is the parents want to know about the child's development and what questions they want answered. The team may then consider these questions during the course of the interview and return to them at the end, either to answer them as well as possible or to discuss what procedures should be adopted to move towards an answer.

The rest of the interview may proceed variously but should contain information about the present situation, what led up to this situation and any progress or deterioration during that time. Where possible the interviewer should try to follow the lead given by the family rather than imposing his or her own structure. It may take longer to follow-up these comments and move the discussion on but generally it will mean they are more relaxed about the whole procedure. It is often difficult to remember exact dates and timespans, particularly when there are several children in the family. Where it is important to record the information as accurately as possible, then it may be necessary to allow time to establish relevant matters surrounding the questions under consideration. A short discussion between the partners may help clear up a time or date as it may have been related to a more memorable family event.

Some clinicians prefer to start with the present situation and work back to early history, and others start at the beginning and work towards the present. Either way is quite acceptable, but it is important to remember that recent events may be fresher in the memory and help to establish links to past events. The process of case-history taking should be a shared one. During its course it is not just the professionals who will have learned something. The family too may begin to see a pattern emerge in the child's development which allows them to make some discoveries about the child's strengths and progress to date. This is very valuable when the child has a complex problem which can seem overwhelming and within which there seems to be little that appears positive. Here are some of the things which may be included in a case-history discussion:

1. Understanding the present situation:
    (a) a description of what the child is like now;
    (b) work through a typical day and what usually happens;
    (c) how the child copes with everyday activities;
    (d) the present input from professionals;
    (e) the present family structure and relationships;

(f) the facilities presently used by the family, whether these are helpful or not;

(g) the family's present understanding of the child's needs;

(h) a description of the child's preferred method of communication.

2. Understanding the past:

    (a) how the family situation became established:

        (i)   the size of the family;

        (ii)   the family dynamics;

        (iii) any previous history of developmental problems in other family members;

        (iv)   how the family functions, the burden of care, other family anxieties;

    (b) the child's story:

        (i)   the history of the pregnancy and birth;

        (ii)   the early developmental history with an emphasis on early communication development;

        (iii) any history of medical problems, childhood illnesses, significant hospitalisations;

        (iv)   depending on the age of the child, the transition to school or other group;

        (v)   the child's social relationships.

3. Looking for progress or deterioration:

    (a) the order and rate at which the child passed the usual developmental milestones (smiling, sitting, walking, babble, words etc.);

    (b) the skills that the child has acquired in the last 6 months;

    (c) any suggestion that the child is not making progress now, or period of static development in the past;

    (d) any suggestion that the child lost skills in the past;

    (e) any suggestion that the child's abilities appear to fluctuate;

    (f) any events related to static or deteriorating development, both social, emotional and medical;

    (g) the child's rate of development in relation to siblings and peers, and parental expectation.

Where the case history is taken by one person, it is clear that they cannot be an expert in all these areas of development. Thus some sections of the case history will be understandably brief and may need supplementing at a later stage. Where the case history is taken in a group situation, it should be possible to include the questions and observations of others where relevant.

Sometimes the information obtained at interview is supplemented by letters and reports from other professionals, particularly where the child comes for a second opinion. Where these are available they should be evaluated carefully in order to see if they provide further evidence in any of the above categories. Equally the parents may have previously made a statement, either informally or formally, about the child's development which is available for discussion. There will be occasions when the parent(s) prefer to give a long monologue, setting out the situation from their perspective. Although this might appear to interfere with a neatly prescribed framework of case-history taking, it should not necessarily be dismissed as neurotic and hysterical nonsense. Parents often feel that the professionals have not heard what they said about the child, and this means that the clinical relationship begins in a very unsatisfactory manner. Case 7 is the story of a 10-year-old boy with a language disorder, as told by his mother.

Case 7

'He seemed normal for the first 2 years of his life. He was always very active and reached all his usual milestones early. It was at about 2 years old that we began to think he had some problems understanding what we said and in expressing himself. He had his hearing tested and that showed that he had 'glue ears'. He had grommets put in for that. In all he had grommets three times over the next few years. He first saw a speech therapist when he was 2½ years old. He seemed to have a very short attention span and difficulty recognising colours, although he could see alright.

'By the time he was 3 years we were very anxious about him. Although he could answer obvious questions, there were times when he didn't seem to hear or understand what we said. I found it very difficult to cope and my GP referred me to a psychiatrist. I was on tranquillisers for quite a while. He was a very friendly boy, very loving to us in the family. He had some funny little ways of communicating and a special little ritual for saying 'hello' which we all had to do. When he was 4 years we referred him to the educational psychologist, and he was finally seen when he was 5 years old. He seemed to puzzle everyone. First of all he was diagnosed as deaf, but he did seem to hear quite a lot of things. He always played quite normally though often on his own. His main problem seemed to be that he didn't understand what people said. Our GP referred us to a paediatrician for a second opinion and that doctor told us the problem was to do with additives in his food. At the time it seemed quite a good idea and we did try an additive-free diet for a while. I don't think it made any difference in the long run.

'He was beginning to get more anxious himself, especially in new situations and his understanding had not improved. The educational psychologist hadn't done anything, and so when he was 6 years old we asked to see the school doctor. The school asked for some extra help for him but this was turned down. He was trying very hard to understand what people said and to make us understand. He would often ask us what people said or what they meant. He was always asking questions although they often sounded a bit funny, like 'What's red mean?'. Finally I went to the local library and read all the books I could find about children's development. I made the diagnosis of receptive language disorder myself. He was 8 years old.

'Our ear, nose and throat (ENT) surgeon referred us for a further assessment to the speech therapist, as his hearing was normal. We waited 16 months for the assessment, then all the speech therapist did was a test and said he had trouble with understanding. We knew that; we wanted someone to suggest what should be done next. Six months later the educational psychologist saw him again and said he was a slow learner but that he was not slow enough to go to a special school or have extra help. We managed to arrange for him to have 20 minutes of speech therapy a week, but the speech therapist was also baffled. She didn't know if the language difficulty was caused by his attention problem or his hearing problem. This was not very encouraging; it was still being described as a hearing problem, although the ENT surgeon said his hearing was normal. The speech therapist thought we should see a teacher for the deaf. He is now 10 years old and although he is rather anxious, especially in new situations, he still attends normal school and gets no other help. He likes computers and copes with his problems in understanding by asking lots of questions. He tends to comprehend what you say literally, and therefore often misses the point. He is not confident, often can't think of the words to say and still requires careful explanations both at home and school. However, he is very happy at home within the family and we love him very much.'

Do not make the mistake of thinking that this is an isolated case. Children with language disorders do have complex problems. The purpose of hearing the history is to try to piece together the whole picture so that effective action can be taken, in the hope that a situation like the one outlined above may not occur.

Other investigations

After taking the case history, we can move on to the next steps. The case-history information, itself, must be carefully evaluated for signs that might suggest further investigations or be direct pointers to diagnosis. In the story in Case 7, the question of the child's hearing obviously needs further investigation. As we shall see, it is not unusual for children with receptive language problems to be described as deaf. Nor is it unusual for them to have 'glue ear', because it is a common childhood condition (and more properly called secretory otitis media – see Appendix I). Among the range of other investigations that may be required, and that will require the expertise of other members of the multidisciplinary team, are the following.

Hearing test

The method used will depend on age. Distraction testing is the usual primary procedure under 2 years old. Where distraction testing fails to establish a threshold and concern is still evident, an electrical test of hearing, such as the auditory evoked potentials (a measure of hearing thresholds at the cerebral level using electronic equipment and often requiring a small child to be sedated) may be used. Above 2 years of age, it should be possible to condition the majority of children and test using free-field audiometry. Between 3 and 4 years, the child should be able to move on to using headphones to complete a pure-tone audiogram. The function of the middle ear and the compliance of the tympanic membrane can be tested using an impedance audiometer. This helps to establish the presence of fluid in the middle ear for the diagnosis of otitis media. Visual inspection of the ear drum by using an auroscope in the ear canal, called otoscopy, will establish whether the ear drum is patent.

Examination of fine and gross motor skills

This may be carried out formally by physio- and occupational therapists or more informally as part of a general developmental check-up. Some expressive language problems are known to have a motor component and language disorders can co-occur with motor disorders like muscular dystrophy (see Appendix I).

Physical examination including neurological examination

A thorough physical examination will be important to establish the presence of signs of particular syndromes or known conditions, even though these are fairly uncommon. The examination usually begins with the skin to see if there are any patches of pigment or unusual birthmarks. Of particular interest are the café-au-lait spots and patches that might indicate neurofibromatosis (see Appendix I) or port wine stains on the face which can be associated with the Sturge–Weber syndrome (also see Appendix I). Some syndromes are recognised from particular facial characteristics, such as Down's syndrome and Williams' syndrome (see Appendix I). The arms and legs should be examined for the presence of hemiplegia or signs of muscular dystrophy. The teeth and the mouth should also be examined. Some conditions, such as incontinentia pigmenti, affect the teeth (see Appendix I). The significance of some of these oral anomalies, including tongue tie, for future speech development remains controversial. Persistent dribbling is a feature of some expressive language problems, the Worster-Drought syndrome and some types of cerebral palsy (see Appendix I). Testing the cranial nerves will reveal any evidence of visual field defects, squints and other ocular anomalies, facial palsy and velopharyngeal incompetence. Measurement of the head circumference should be compared to the well established norms so that microcephaly or hydrocephaly may be ruled out. Both of these conditions can have a significant effect on developmental progress.

Medical investigations and tests

The examination may indicate the benefit of further investigations or tests. The simplest of these may be a blood test. However, for some children having a blood test is an unpleasant experience, and it is rarely necessary to do this on the first visit. Even if the child has come a long distance, most of the routine blood tests which screen for common developmental syndromes can be carried out locally. One of the blood tests may include an examination of chromosomes. Whilst most children with well-known chromosomal abnormalities, such as Down's syndrome, are diagnosed within the newborn period, other syndromes are less common and thus may not be diagnosed until later when the child's developmental progress does not appear to be normal. At present there is no one blood test that confirms the presence of language disorder. However, some of the conditions which can co-occur with language disorder should be investigated as they may have a significant effect on the prognosis, both for the individual child and for other family members. These include Duchenne muscular dystrophy (the children usually die in their teens) and the fragile X syndrome (see Appendix I), which may be part of a wider condition affecting other aspects of cognitive development.

Unless the child is suspected of having a specific cerebral lesion (from the presence of a hemiplegia or visual field defect), a computed tomography (CT) scan of the brain is unlikely to show any useful information in the child who presents with language disorder and no other signs. Where the measurement of the head circumference indicates a head size considered abnormally large and not consistent with the rest of the family, it may be used to rule out hydrocephalus. Otherwise, we shall probably have to wait for the new generation of brain scanning techniques to become more widely used before we can see whether they are useful in contributing to our understanding of the cerebral mechanisms of language disorder. Where velopharyngeal incompetence is suspected helpful investigations include lateral cine radiograph, videofluoroscopic radiograph and nasal endoscopy.

Assessment of general cognitive function

Once again this may be informal, within the framework of a general developmental check-up, or a more formal psychological assessment. The Stycar Sequences by Sheridan (1973) are the most commonly used and simplest framework for assessing general development. They provide a description of the normal sequence of development from birth to 5 years in four developmental areas: posture and gross movements, vision and fine movements, hearing and speech, social behaviour, and play. Other developmental schedules in common use include the Griffiths Scales (Griffiths, 1954, 1970). The scale for babies to 2 years is the older of the two (1954) and was extended in 1970 to include children up to 8 years. Six areas of development are tested in a range of activities: locomotor, personal and social, hearing and speech, hand and eye coordination, performance tests, and practical reasoning. The measures are standardised on British children and a developmental quotient can be obtained for each scale. The average of these quotients equals the child's general intelligence quotient.

There is a vast range of psychological assessment available. Traditionally the Wechsler Intelligence Scale for Children – Revised edition (WISC-R; Wechsler, 1974) has been popular and many research studies quote it. It is suitable for children aged 6–15 years and is divided into performance and verbal items. A full IQ score as well as separate performance and verbal IQs can therefore be obtained. There are six performance and six verbal subtests. To carry out the performance items, the child does not need to use any spoken language. The performance subtests are timed and the child is credited the more quickly an item is completed. Other assessments seek to produce a psychological test which requires the minimum knowledge of language for its completion, so as not to put the language-impaired child at a disadvantage. One of these is the Leiter International Performance Scale (Leiter, 1969) which is totally non-verbal (no verbal instructions or responses). It is therefore particularly useful with the deaf or language-disordered child. It is suitable for children from 2 years old, and it involves a range of matching tasks. At the simplest level the child is asked to match colour or shape (one dimension only). As the test progresses the child must match increasingly complex items with two or three dimensions being considered (e.g. shape, colour, number, size). In this way the test becomes increasingly difficult with the incorporation of finer perceptual distinctions and more abstract relations between the items.

Some of these psychological assessments can be very lengthy. Where a shorter, and obviously less comprehensive, measure is required the Goodenough–Harris Drawing Test (Harris, 1963) may be considered. This is a simple drawing task in which the children are asked to draw either a man or woman or themselves. The style in which it is executed and the number of items included in the drawing can be related to age norms to give a measure of each child's maturity. The test covers the age range 3–13 years (norms from the USA) and there is a possible total score of 50 marks. Items 1–8 are concerned with the gross details of the head, legs and trunk etc. Items 9–17 are for facial details, such that 12 marks the presence of a nose, 13 the mouth and 14 both the mouth and nose. When the drawing is in profile the lips must be modelled correctly and, if in two dimensions, then two lips must be shown, not just one line. Details of clothing are considered in items 18–22 and 23–35 are for the fine details of the body form, like the fingers, thumbs, elbows and heels. The fine degree of motor coordination used to execute the drawing is considered in items 36–41; for example, item 38 considers the regularity of the head outline such that it should be better than a primitive circle or ellipse and the lines should be firm and meet together smoothly. Finally, items 42–50 deal with very fine detail of the ears, eyes, facial expression, chin, forehead and correct profile details. Examples of such figures drawn by children are shown in Figure 3.1.

This is not a comprehensive list of possible ways of evaluating the language-impaired child's general and cognitive development. Many experienced professionals will have their own preferred methods. The contribution of longitudinal observations made by the parents, playgroup leader, portage worker or teacher should not be overlooked when considering the learning potential of a language-impaired child.

The questions the parents originally voiced must remain a major influence in the diagnostic procedure. One most commonly asked is about the cause of the problem. The parents may have expended much time and anxiety searching the history and their own conduct for a reason for the child's problem. Excessive guilt is rarely helpful in moving forward to effective management. However, as the above list indicates, establishing the cause of a child's language impairment is rarely straightforward. In the child with no significant events in early history or family history and with normal developmental progress in all other respects, including normal hearing and no neurological signs, it is often not possible to establish a cause. This does not mean that the diagnostic procedure is useless; it has an important value in ruling out other significant problems. It does indicate our ignorance about the origins of language disorder and the need for continued research in this field.

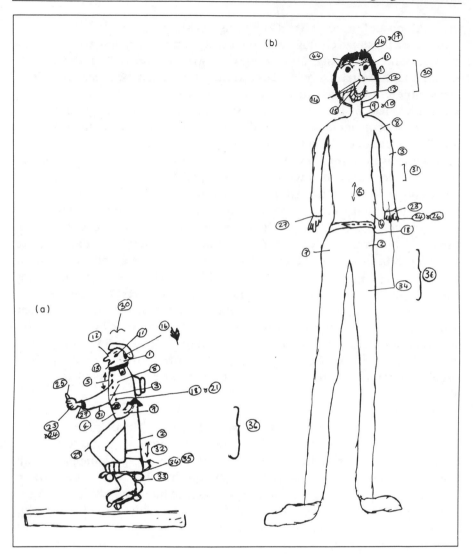

Figure 3.1 (a) Goodenough–Harris Draw-a-Man Test: example by a child of 7;11 years, who had a total score of 26 and an age-equivalent score of 9 years. (b) Example by a child aged 8;1 years, who had a total score of 26 and an age-equivalent score of 9 years

Language assessment

Within the multidisciplinary team, the speech therapist's major role is to determine the nature and extent of the child's language problem. How this is done will depend on the age of the child, the time available and the amount of relevant previous information he or she has access to. Where this is the first time the child has been seen by a speech therapist, he or she will be starting from scratch. It is therefore unlikely that all the necessary information will be obtained in one assessment period. This is also true where the child is very young (under 2;6 years). This period of any child's development is crucial and changeable and it may be necessary to re-evaluate a provisional diagnosis at a later stage. Where the therapist is working single-handed, it is probably unreasonable to expect to get through case history and initial assessment in one interview without the family, child and therapist showing the strain of such an intensive encounter. It is much better to plan to continue the assessment on another occasion when the situation will be more familiar to the child and everyone will feel fresher.

Within the team situation the assessment can be carried out in several ways. Some people favour taking the child (with or without other family members) to another less distracting or quieter room for the language assessment. In a centre with two-way viewing facilities, the other professionals and family members can still watch what is taking place and therefore be able to discuss this later. Others find it satisfactory to carry out the language assessment in the same room as the previous interview. This saves continually moving around and introducing the child to another new environment. Whichever method is chosen, the most important factor is that the family and other professionals can continue to contribute to the assessment procedure by their observations. Some clinicians find this idea rather intimidating and prefer to take the child off on their own, reporting back to the group later. Experience suggests that the amount of information and support gained from the assessment being observed by others is too great to let personal insecurities dictate the separatist approach.

Before starting the assessment, the therapist should review the information available so far, particularly from the case history. Where time is at a premium, this will help to ensure that the therapist chooses, as far as possible, the 'right' assessment. Where other information, perhaps from previous assessments, is available, this should also be carefully evaluated. Some formal assessments cannot be repeated within a certain timespan without impinging on their validity. Where the timespan is sufficient, a repeat assessment will make it possible for a direct comparison to be made, which is one way of measuring progress. Where informal observations are available, they may indicate whether the child is ready for formal assessment or give the therapist an indication of further avenues not previously explored.

A full discussion of the ways in which a child's language can be assessed is given in Chapter 2. It will not be repeated here. This discussion will concentrate on how to establish a baseline for the child's language skills which can:

1. Establish severity.
2. Recommend areas requiring treatment.
3. Be repeated over time to establish the natural history and prognosis of
   the disorder.

The therapist should aim to produce as comprehensive a profile of the
child's language as the circumstances allow. It will be necessary to sample
as many skills as possible. If the child is not yet ready for formal assessment,
then this will need to be done within an informal framework (see Chapter
2 for some suggestions of how to do this). For the older child, some formal
measures may also be introduced. It is important to get the balance right
and to finish by inquiring whether the family feels that the child has given a
good, average or poor performance according to what they would expect.
Many people are suspicious of assessment procedures. This gives them a
chance to say how they felt the child managed and is part of the learning
process that assessment is for all of us, families and professionals alike.

It seems sensible to give an example of how a language profile might be
established during the kind of assessment we have been discussing. This is
a tried and tested method used over a number of years within a
multidisciplinary team; it does not pretend to be fully comprehensive but it
does fulfil the criteria listed above. It works best with those aged 4–12
years who have come for at least a second opinion, where some previous
information is already available and where the child can cooperate with
formal testing. It aims to sample the following areas of language ability (the
individual tests are discussed in more detail in Chapter 2).

Auditory–verbal comprehension

The Test for Reception of Grammar (TROG; Bishop, 1983) is the first
choice as it is well structured, easy to carry out, appealing to children and
careful analysis gives much information. If the child is not able to cope with
this, then either the Derbyshire Comprehension Test or the Comprehension Scale of the Reynell Scale may be used. With practice the TROG can be
administered to children aged 3;9 years and over, but if only one or two
sections are passed it gives little information and it is better to use one of
the other tests in such circumstances.

Word-finding and lexical organisation

The Test of Word Finding (TWF; German, 1986) is a very comprehensive
way of investigating a child's naming ability and lexical organisation skills.
However, many will not yet be familiar with it. The Word Finding
Vocabulary Test (WFVT; Renfew, 1972c) is simple and quick to administer
and recently new norms have been produced. When using this one it can
be supplemented with the Auditory Association subtest of the Illinois Test

of Psycholinguistic Ability (ITPA; Kirk, McCarthy and Kirk, 1968) to give a broader view of lexical organisation skills (the TWF already includes such a subtest).

Auditory–verbal memory and discrimination

A sentence repetition test and an auditory discrimination test are useful for this section. The Spreen–Benton Sentence Repetition Test has norms for children 6–13 years (Gaddes and Crockett, 1975). Although young children may be reluctant to do sentence repetition, this one is better than most as the sentence length only increases by one syllable each time. Auditory discrimination may be carried out informally with lists of minimal pairs which the child has to listen to and judge as the same or different.

Expressive language

An extensive sample of expressive language may be unrealistic, and there may never be sufficient time to analyse it anyway. Ten sentences may be sufficient to demonstrate a pattern in sentence construction, in which case the Action Picture Test (Renfew, 1977a) is quick and simple. A story-telling method can be a useful way to obtain a language sample. Renfrew's (1972b) Bus Story works on this principle and has been found to be useful in predicting prognosis (Bishop and Edmundson, 1987). For those who prefer a different kind of story, without picture cues, the story-telling method recommended by Mandler and Johnson (1977) can be recommended (detailed in Appendix II). Unfortunately, no norms are available for this, but a helpful overview of the child's communicative competence can be obtained. Children without language problems from the age of 6 upwards can do this satisfactorily.

Looking at the results from a group of tests can be confusing; they can be analysed at so many different levels. When adding up the score according to the test manual, there may be the choice of converting to an age equivalent or a standard score, or expressing it in terms of the centile level. The choice will depend on what kind of interpretation is required. For those who prefer to follow the idea that all language disorder is really language delay, an age equivalent score may be a more comfortable interpretation. It reinforces the notion that the child is just rather slower, perhaps a year or so behind his or her chronological age. It is rarely helpful when considering management as it also reinforces the notion that the child is really just immature and should be treated as a younger child. This generally leads to a lower level of language being supplied, and to social and cognitive expectations also being lowered. If the child is aged 6 then why treat her or him as a 5 year old? It is much better to recognise that there is a mismatch between the child's language ability and other areas of skills that needs specific attention. It is also usually more helpful to see the child as part of a peer group; this is where centile scores can be useful. They provide an idea of where the child is in terms of the normal range at that age. Thus, we can see if the child is likely to be able to keep up with peers in a mixed class or be at a serious disadvantage linguistically, cognitively and socially.

When trying to make a comparison across tests, the z-score is a useful interpretation. However, not all test scores can be readily converted to z-scores. This will depend on what information is available in the manual. When converting to z-scores a calculator is recommended because it is a laborious calculation to do otherwise. The z-score is calculated as follows:

$$z\text{-score} = \frac{\text{Raw score} - \text{Mean score}}{\text{Standard deviation}}$$

The raw score refers to the actual score the child achieved. The mean score is the average score for children at that age. The standard deviation is probably the most commonly used expression of the variance within a normally distributed sample to be used in test manuals. The following example demonstrates how this calculation looks in practice. A child of 4;3 years scores a total of five blocks passed on the TROG. This would be converted to a z-score as follows:

$$z\text{-score} = \frac{5 - 8}{3.5} = -0.85$$

This score would fall at the low end of the normal range, which is between -1 and $+1$.

If it is possible to convert the test scores available to z-scores, then any mismatch between particular areas of language skill tested will be revealed, e.g. a child aged 5 years who has the following z-scores:

TROG	− 0.5
WFVT	− 2.5
Auditory Association	− 1.2

(These tests are discussed in detail in Chapter 2.)

These scores suggest a severe word-finding difficulty, with normal verbal comprehension in which the ability to recall words by association is much better than confrontational naming. In turn it would suggest a possible treatment strategy which, capitalising on the good verbal comprehension, gradually helps the child to generate his or her own cues to aid word finding. The way in which such a programme would be constructed would depend on further qualitative analysis of the test data to discover what, if any, cueing strategies help the child.

The analysis of test results does not end with a row of figures. Whilst they do make a statement about severity, it is qualitative analysis which moves us on to determining treatment strategies. In some tests a pattern will emerge of the items the child passes or fails. In others it will be possible to determine what strategies the child uses to help her- or himself succeed. There is no such thing as a random response on a test; such a conclusion probably means that the pattern has not been fully investigated. If using the kind of test battery recommended above, some of the test manuals give suggestions for qualitative analysis. The TROG manual includes an analysis of grammatical vs lexical errors to help determine whether the child has specific difficulties with certain grammatical structures or a more general comprehension problem. The TWF includes an analysis of the types of cues which aided the child's naming. If a test does not contain such information, then it does not rule out the possibility of qualitative analysis. Porch (1972) included some of the basic requirements of a qualitative analysis in his Porch Index of Communicative Ability in Children (PICAC). Whilst many feel that a 16-point code to determine the quality of response is rather excessive, the principle remains sound. It is possible to draw up a personal code which incorporates the basics, including speed, completeness and accuracy of response. Such a code may quickly be noted during the assessment and then analysed later. Here is an example of the kind of code which could be used with TROG:

1. All accurate and complete responses not requiring a repetition or cue will not receive any additional annotation.
2. All complete and accurate responses carried out after a delay of up to 10 seconds (not formally measured) will be coded as B.
3. All complete and accurate responses carried out after the tester repeats the instructions will be coded as C.
4. All complete and accurate responses carried out after the child requests a repetition will be coded as C(i).
5. All responses which are complete and accurate after the child initially chooses another response and then changes his or her mind (a self-corrected response) will be coded as D.

This is not the only way of coding such responses but it has proved useful in the analysis of receptive language problems in a group of children with acquired childhood aphasia (Lees, 1989) and in the diagnosis of language-impaired children within the multidisciplinary team previously discussed. It is the kind of code which could easily be applied to other tests.

Analysing these qualitative responses is not straightforward as conclusions are to some extent subjective and open to other interpretation. Few test manuals consider the place of qualitative analysis and therefore fail to give normal data on, for example, speed of response or the number of repetitions required. However, where a clear pattern emerges, it may be possible to suggest that a child appears to rely on a need for repetition in verbal comprehension tasks or particular kinds of cues in naming tasks. These are helpful observations when formulating preliminary hypotheses for treatment programmes. They are also helpful in providing initial ideas to discuss with family and teachers about how to cope with the language problem in the everyday situation. If repetition or cueing helps then use it, at least as an interim measure. A remedial strategy can then be built on success rather than on failure.

Summary of the diagnostic procedures

1. Take a detailed case history, particularly of early communication development.
2. Begin to draw up a series of formal and informal observations of the child's communication skills.
3. Liaise with other professionals concerned with the child's development.
4. Establish a baseline of the child's language difficulties against which progress can be determined.
5. Initiate the further assessment of the child by other professionals or a multidisciplinary team for further investigation and assessment if necessary.
6. Look for strengths and weaknesses in the child's language profile which could be used in the planning of an intervention programme.
7. Continue to evaluate the child's progress, by formal and informal measures, and alter the intervention programme as necessary.

One of the most common questions asked by parents of language-impaired children at assessment is about prognosis; they want to know if the child will get better. Our knowledge of the natural history of language impairment is by no means comprehensive. Equally it is a question that requires long-term observation in order to be answered with any degree of certainty. One assessment is hardly likely to be sufficient on which to base an informed opinion that the child 'will grow out of it in 2 years time' for example. If previous observations of the child are available and some indication of a familial pattern of development which includes language disorder, these can be very useful in answering the question of prognosis. A comprehensive language profile, as discussed above, can also be compared with other known patterns of language disorder as a guide to determining prognosis.

It is possible to begin to answer the question of prognosis if reference is made to other research findings (see particularly Bishop and Edmundson, 1987), other known patterns of language impairment (like those proposed by Rapin and Allen, 1987) and the child's previous history. Where previous test results are available, they can be used to document the child's progress

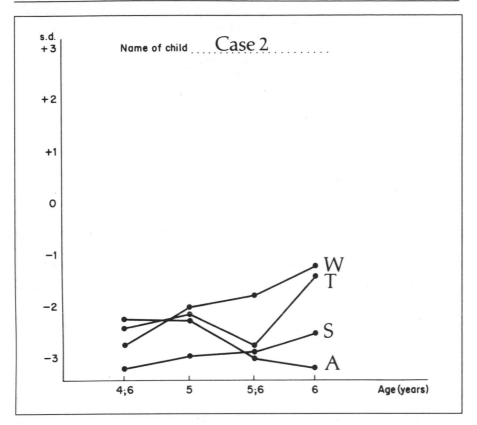

Figure 3.2 Language profile graph of Case 2. T = Test for Reception of Grammar; W = Word Finding Vocabulary Test; S = Sentence Repetition; A = Association Naming

to date and therefore establish any emerging trend. Some examples of this approach for acquired childhood aphasia are given in Chapter 9. The same thing can be done with developmental language disorder, although of course there will be no point of actual onset as in acquired childhood aphasia. Figure 3.2 shows the test results of the language-disordered child described in Case 2 taken over several assessments. When graphs like this are made of the progress children make, it is possible to evaluate whether it is a gradual or sudden progress, where other events and blocks of treatment occur in relation to the progress made, and whether there are any plateaus or periods of negative progress. Although acquired childhood aphasia has been considered a rare disorder in childhood, careful analysis of case histories and patterns of development in language-impaired children over a number of years has confirmed the view that deterioration, developmental arrest and plateau are common features in the early lives of many language-impaired children.

A graph of a child's progress over time can also help to answer questions

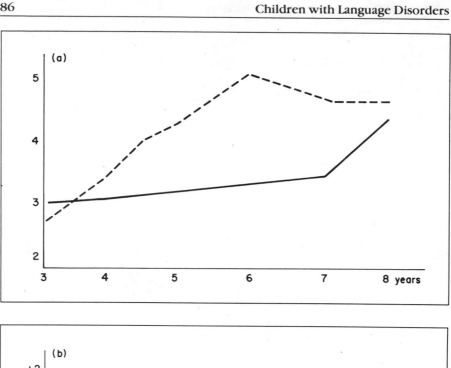

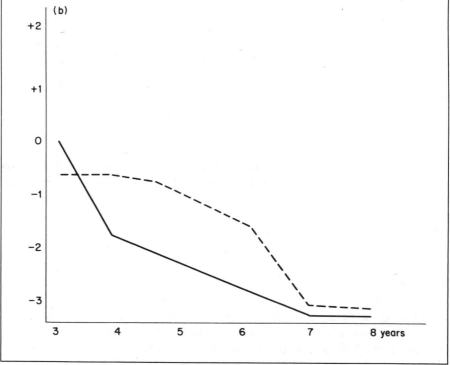

Figure 3.3 Assessment of verbal comprehension (− − −) and expressive language (———) using RDLS for Case 8. (a) Age-equivalent scores; (b) standard scores

about the child in relation to peer group, which may be an important consideration for educational placement. However, the information obtained may vary depending on how the results are shown. Figure 3.3 shows the graphs for Case 8 and demonstrates the different information that can be obtained depending on the way test scores are displayed.

Case 8

A child of 8 years with a language disorder was seen because concern was being voiced about his deteriorating language skills. He was in a class in a mainstream primary school, and both his teacher and speech therapist felt that his performance had shown deterioration over the course of the previous two terms. Neurological examination showed no evidence of degenerative disease or active epilepsy. Examination of previous results using the RDLS with scores converted to age equivalents (the most commonly used method) did suggest that he was continuing to make progress. Since the age of 3;3 years when first tested, he had improved from an age-equivalent score for expressive language of 3;3 years (normal for his age) to one of 4;6 years (now over 3 years behind his age). Similarly with verbal comprehension which had progressed from 2;10 at 3;3 years to 4;6 at 8 years. However, an analysis of these results using a standard score interpretation quickly demonstrated that the progress he had made over that time was insufficient to ensure that he kept abreast of his peers: he was falling further and further away from the mean score, and this was being perceived as deterioration. This situation required that some provision be made for his special educational needs.

Treating or Managing the Problem from the Baseline

Having established the diagnosis and the baseline of the language problem, it is possible to use this as a point from which to evaluate the effects of treatment. A fuller account of the methodology behind a single case research design is given in Chapter 8. In the everyday clinical situation, it is important to remember that, although progress can be measured from a one-point baseline, a treatment effect will be shown more clearly where more baseline points are available. In the main we will want to evaluate the effects of language therapy and/or educational placement. This will also require longitudinal observations of the child's response to a variety of informal situations which cannot be measured by test scores alone. These include the child's integration into the peer group, the child's relationships

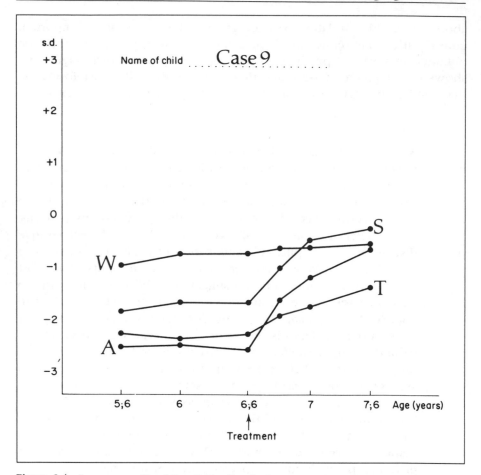

Figure 3.4 Language profile of Case 9. T = Test for Reception of Grammar; W = Word Finding Vocabulary Test; S = Sentence Repetition; A = Association Naming

with individual adults and children, and the child's effective communication both with individuals and within the group. However, a baseline which uses test results can give some indication of specific areas of progress, remembering that the aim is not to treat to the test score but to achieve communicative competence. Figure 3.4 shows a graph for Case 9 and indicates where the period of treatment began in relation to changes in test scores.

Case 9

A boy, 6 years old, had a language disorder of long standing. He was well known to speech therapy services, but it had not previously

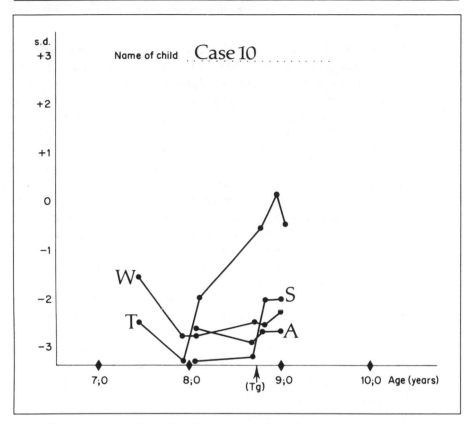

Figure 3.5   Language profile of Case 10. T = Test for Reception of Grammar; W = Word Finding Vocabulary Test; S = Sentence Repetition; A = Association Naming; Tg = anticonvulsant

proved possible to arrange a more specific and intensive treatment for his severe language problems. Figure 3.4 shows how his auditory verbal processing, grammatical comprehension, and semantic association showed gradual improvement when a more intensive and specific programme aimed at these receptive language difficulties was introduced at the age of 6;6 years. This amounted to three blocks of therapy, each of 2 weeks' duration, over 6 months, with a return to once weekly therapy in between the blocks.

Sometimes the treatment to be evaluated is not language therapy. Occasionally it may be necessary to monitor what effect the treatment given by another professional has on the child's language development. This point is illustrated in Case 10 and Figure 3.5.

Case 10

This boy was referred at the age of 8 years for further investigations as there was some concern that his language skills, particularly his verbal comprehension, might be fluctuating. He had a congenital left hemiplegia arising from a large infarct in the region of the right middle cerebral artery and affecting a major part of the right motor cortex (confirmed by CT scan). He had no history of epilepsy or other developmental problems. He had first been seen by a speech therapist at the age of 2;6 years concerning his speech and language development. Although he had made some progress with this, he continued to have a severe language problem and had been placed in a language unit since the age of 5. His mother said that she had often been concerned about his hearing in the past and that he frequently appeared not to hear. However, all hearing tests were, and always had been, normal. Test scores of receptive language obtained since the age of 2;11 years, using the RDLS and later the TROG, consistently gave standard scores below −2. Apart from the motor signs on the left consistent with the hemiplegia, there were no other neurological signs. An EEG revealed an epileptic focus in the left temporal lobe, the region associated with the auditory association cortex and Wernicke's area. Anticonvulsant medication (carbamazepine) was begun and the dose gradually increased until blood tests confirmed a level within the recommended therapeutic range. Repeat language testing did suggest an improvement in receptive language. Only long-term follow-up will confirm whether this is maintained.

It is not possible to say that this type of intervention is always effective in fluctuating receptive language disorders. The subject is discussed more fully in Chapter 9. The major emphasis is on the role that language assessment may have in monitoring the effectiveness of the use of anticonvulsants in children with language disorder and epilepsy.

The History and Implications of the Condition

Language disorders can have a life-time effect. What begins as a history of 'late talking' may eventually become a long-term difficulty with verbal communication which affects all aspects of life: employment, education, social integration. Whilst many parents begin with the question 'Will he or she grow out of it?', others come to understand its long-term implications very gradually. Reviewing the history of the condition with the parents, and careful discussion of the results of language tests and other investigations, is vital for an opportunity to come to terms with the implications. Again, one member of the team may be more skilled in this area than others. Equally it may take more than one visit to fully discuss all the information to the parents' satisfaction. It is a process which cannot be rushed but needs to be handled sensitively so that all parties get the feeling of progress rather than one of going round and round in circles. The professionals involved also need to understand their own feelings as they impinge on their clinical effectiveness. It is not uncommon for feelings of defensiveness or suspicion to accompany any suggestion by the parents that they would like to seek further opinion. However, frank opposition to such a suggestion is likely only to lead to a breakdown in the relationship with the family. It is not unreasonable for the family to wish to 'leave no stone unturned' in the search for a more positive prognosis for their child. Rather than opposition, support is usually more productive. Where possible, this should include liaison with those who will provide the second opinion. The results of a clinical picture built up over time are not meant to influence them to adopt a particular view. Rather, such results contribute to the long-term perspective which an individual assessment cannot provide. Where the second opinion provides a different perspective from the one originally offered, it is important for all concerned to carefully evaluate the evidence which has led to this rather than to adopt immediately a defensive position. Enough emphasis cannot be placed on how important the views of fellow professionals are in establishing an accurate diagnosis. As for discussing management, in a complex case, this also benefits from a broad view, not in order to negate previous attempts but to support appropriate forward planning.

Recognising the Condition when it recurs

In evaluating the risk of the recurrence of language disorder among siblings of the affected child, Robinson (1987) reports figures ranging from 1:4.5 to 1:5.2 with brothers being more at risk than sisters (between 1:3.7 to 1:4.4). Some recent attempts to chart the occurrence of language disorder in extended families has met with some success. Where the language problem is associated with another developmental disorder, its identification may have other important implications. Syndromes which are manifest in early childhood may be terminal before adulthood (e.g. Duchenne muscular dystrophy). Others can be associated with a progressively worsening condition, like some types of epilepsy. Where anxiety about the genetic implications of the condition cannot be answered by the professionals available, then genetic counselling may be the next step. This will allow the parents to discuss the situation both in respect of further pregnancies for themselves and future generations of the family.

The Research Implications of Differential Diagnosis

Differential diagnosis and long-term follow-up is a useful part of clinically based research initiatives to understand further language disorder. It is, after all, the families and professionals working with the child who need to know what the outcome is likely to be. Differential diagnosis can help to establish patterns within the clinical population which can form a useful basis for comparison. However, not all professionals will be working in teams or have sufficient clinical experience behind them to allow them to establish the diagnoses that have been discussed here. Recent attempts to make comprehensive diagnostic procedures more readily available to isolated or less experienced clinicians through the availability of computer technology has led to the development of so-called 'expert systems'. To date these have been experimental and available to a few doctors, for example in the area of the diagnosis of infection (Fox, Alvey and Myers, 1983). Trying to devise an expert system for the differential diagnosis of language disorder is not easy as there are a large number of variables to consider. Equally, some are sceptical that it is possible to make such a diagnosis from written information alone (i.e. without actually seeing the child). An experimental version of an expert system to diagnose language disorder has recently been described and provisionally tested by Dalton (1989); further work is in progress which uses the Rapin and Allen (1987) six categories as the basis for the diagnostic criteria and presents these via a computer screen in a range of 'user friendly' choices. The key features of the six subtypes are also presented in checklist form as a second line for borderline cases or for those where information is incomplete so that the user knows what to look for next. Whilst it is not yet ready for extensive clinical trials, it does provide some initial impetus in this area. Experience working with the system has proved valuable in further crystallising ideas about differential diagnosis, particularly how to describe logically and clearly the features of language disorder so they can be understood by others. It has also provided further constructive criticism of the Rapin and Allen model.

In conclusion, this chapter has explored the advantages of differential diagnosis, particularly within a multidisciplinary setting, for the management of the language-disordered child. Having discussed the way in which it can help to establish the severity of a condition, suggest areas requiring intervention and provide a basis for the discussion of prognosis, we are now ready to move on, in Chapters 4, 5 and 6, to an evaluation of intervention methods which can be used with language-disordered children.

Chapter 4
Treatment and Management of Pre-school Children with Language Disorder

Summary

This chapter concerns the development of individual programmes which include small logical steps. The aim is to create optimum learning environments for language-disordered children. Communication skills are discussed separately in terms of practical problems and solutions. However, the clinical goal is to integrate these skills and generalise knowledge in order that the child becomes a competent language generator.

Introduction

Whilst separating assessment from treatment and management seems appropriate within the context of chapter headings in a book, it is a fairly artificial notion in practice. In the 'real world' they are all part of a continuous process and the question of where assessment ends and treatment begins is not clear cut. It is also not clear whether treatment is necessarily a narrower view than management. Whilst these terms may be open to interpretation (and, after all, what terms are not), there must be some essential agreement on what is being aimed at. Our aims are two-fold:

1. What does the child need to know about language?
2. How can we facilitate this learning?

Clinicians may have part of the answer to the first question after the initial assessment, but a complete and comprehensive answer to them both may be more difficult to assemble. This is particularly true if the child is distractible and uncooperative. In these circumstances it is simply not worth carrying on with endless formal test procedures, which the child continues to fail, only to amass many negative results. Knowing what the child cannot do is not the same thing as discovering how he or she can succeed. Helping the child to succeed is a process that should begin on the first day.

Before an intervention programme can be put into motion, we do need to establish the rationale which lies behind the particular approach we will adopt. The basis of our beliefs about the child's strengths and weaknesses, and how they are formed, developed and changed, will affect the way we approach the individual child. However, the what and why of intervention is continually changing. Twenty years ago the rationale would probably have been based on the theoretical model of the Illinois Test of Psycholinguistic Abilities (ITPA) that language development depended on a number of recognisable skills which could be accurately separated and measured (discussed in Chapter 2). The clinician, having separately measured the strengths and weaknesses of these constituent skills, could then work on each of them in isolation and thus improve the overall language ability. An accompanying programme (GOAL) (Kirk and Kirk, 1971) was designed specifically for this purpose. The children improved on the programme but this did not generalise to overall language performance (Bloom and Lahey, 1978). This notion has therefore been criticised by many researchers (Smith and Marx, 1971; Newcomer et al, 1973) and is not borne out by recent research which is more concerned with the complexity of developing language and language-related skills. Thus, the interaction of these processes rather than their separation is now emphasised (Bowerman, 1982; Chiat and Hirson, 1987).

More recently the emphasis has been on the integration of basic language skills in more natural contexts. An example of this model of treatment is the Derbyshire Language Scheme (DLS) (Knowles and Masidlover, 1982). As previously discussed, the programme contains many excellent ideas for eliciting and introducing language material in a variety of contexts and is well researched. However, the authors do not claim that it is a 'blanket approach' for all types of language problems. Certainly, when faced with a child whose language appears to be developing in an abnormal and bizarre way, and where, initially at least, adult verbal guidance seems to interfere with functioning, the DLS has limited use. In these circumstances it is usually more productive to return to the notions of prerequisite or underlying cognitive skills, such as those outlined in the Wolfson Pre-school Language Programme (Cooper, Moodley and Reynell, 1978). This approach suggests a theoretical relationship between associated language and other cognitive skills that must gradually be integrated so that the child can become a competent language generator (Cooper, Moodley and Reynell, 1978; Reynell, 1980).

The questions which face our appraisal of these and other treatment models include (Leonard, 1979; Ward, 1984; Tallal, Stark and Mellitis, 1985):

1. Exactly what skills are necessary to develop language?
2. Is there a finite number?

3. Can they really be isolated?
4. Even if they can be isolated, can they be measured reliably?
5. How does a problem in one area affect another?
6. If the areas are interrelated, how does treating one aspect affect another?

It is clear that there are many things about language development which we have still to understand. Whilst it is easy to criticise any theoretical framework on the basis of what's missing, what we do not yet know or what has not been reliably proven, we continue to be faced with the clinical dilemma of what to do. Research and clinical practice must work hand in hand to address some of these missing links. Clinicians working with language-disordered children are in a good position to begin to find answers to some of these questions provided that they accurately record and quantify their treatment procedures (see Chapters 7 and 8).

The present state of knowledge is such that there does not appear to be any one method or particular approach which can categorically be said to be better than another. However, an oversimplistic view of intervention should be avoided. For example, it is clear that working on an auditory memory deficit by memorising many series of digits does not equate precisely with the problem of processing complex instructions in the classroom. In practice, most individual treatment programmes will include techniques and ideas from both 'tailor-made' schemes and the clinician's own ideas and equipment. The clinician obviously wants to ensure that the learning situation is as natural as possible, but this does not necessarily mean that any stimulating environment will do. Where the child has a language disorder it is clear that he or she cannot learn in the usual fashion from the natural language environment. Equally, it cannot necessarily be assumed that he or she could learn language any better in an environment that just had more language in it.

When constructing a suitable language environment for the language-disordered child, we need to be prepared to alter or reduce anything in that environment according to the child's responses. We need to consider the basic components of the activities presented in order to discover which factors may be hindering or influencing the child's progress within that activity. Initially, at least, it may be necessary to keep activities as 'pure' as possible, even though our eventual aim is integration of skills. Thus, symbolic play may need to be a non-verbal activity before even the simplest verbal language is added to it. Whilst the eventual aim is integration of skills and their generalisation to new situations, this may sometimes only be achieved in part. However, before dealing with actual ideas and practical suggestions, it would be helpful to deal with a few common misconceptions.

Attention work is the same as 'go games'

A 'go game' is a commonly used device for improving attention and cooperation in distractible preschool children. The name is derived from the way in which the adult instructs the child to perform a simple action by the use of a minimal verbal directive: 'Go!'. For example, using a posting box, the adult may initially help the child to select the correct brick for a particular hole. Then, holding the brick in the child's hand over the hole, say 'go' and encourage the child to release the brick. The adult would then gradually reduce the amount of physical guidance provided for the task as the child's attention and cooperation increased. It should be possible to construct many variations on this type of game such that the basic prerequisites remain. Essentially these are a simple performance task well within the child's ability which requires the child to select and then attend, listening for the verbal command, before completing the task.

It is, of course, an exaggeration to suggest that attention work is limited to games of this kind. Whilst repetition is clearly important for the young language-disordered child, boredom does need to be avoided. Attention control is fundamentally important to language development and does need to be assessed and managed during the first stages of treatment. Early attention work may involve the use of key words or commands which require a simple action and response (as described in the 'go games'). It is also likely that during therapy the child will need directions and help in controlling attention in order to sustain an activity. This may involve the use of key words, like 'listen', 'look' and 'good', by the therapist. These techniques are usually quite effective when dealing with the average language-delayed child, who is immature and distractible, or the preschool child with poor listening skills due to previous or on-going conductive hearing loss, or the preschool child with phonological problems needing listening and attention work. For most children then, the provision of good listening models coupled with some attention work should enable them to pass quickly through the early developmental stages (Reynell, 1980) to arrive at a more appropriate level of attention control, at least for the purposes of language intervention, such as level 3 or even 4 (see Chapter 2). By this stage the important point is that adult verbal guidance is now able to help the child achieve more, so that, within the clinical situation, language direction can be provided by the therapist. Case number 6 (see Chapter 2) is an example of a young language-disordered child requiring listening and attention work.

Case 6

This girl was referred to speech therapy at the age of 3 years by her parents and health visitor. Her mother said of her that 'she talked rubbish and didn't listen'. Her mother expressed a personal concern that this problem was in some way 'her fault', because she had an uncle with a general learning difficulty. Other than this there was no evidence of speech and language problems in the family history. The girl had one older brother whose development had not given cause for concern. Both parents were healthy – the father was an office worker and the mother was not in paid employment. Birth and early developmental history were not remarkable. She was described as a 'gregarious character and full of drama'.

Early work concentrated on the basics of listening, gaining eye contact and inhibiting inappropriate verbal output. It took the first session for her to understand what was required in the basic 'go game'. Initially it was necessary to hold her hands and turn her face to the adult before giving her a command. She would regularly stare anywhere but at the adult's face and wander off in the middle of the task. Her bizarre and repetitive expressive language was reduced considerably over 6 months of intensive therapy, so that statements and questions became more appropriate like: 'I'm getting a bicycle for my birthday!', 'I'm a good girl aren't I?', 'Shelagh, he hit me on my arm'. However, if she was placed in a situation where there was simply too much language and verbal direction, her attention and expressive language content would rapidly deteriorate: 'Oh you silly man, you silly man, chussy chussy, chussy, you silly man aren't you, Daisy, Daisy give me your answer do'. In a structured language environment she was able to respond well and transferred to a mainstream school at the age of 5 years. However, on initial transfer her attention and language skills regressed for about 3 weeks and then regained their former level.

Unfortunately most language-disordered children have poor attention control, which remains vulnerable and can be seriously affected by new learning situations. It is often necessary to consider attention as an integral part of the language programme and to develop many intermediate steps in attention work. In this respect attention work with language-disordered children should not be considered separately from all other aspects of language work but always be incorporated into language programmes. This is particularly true where new material is introduced. Some basic attention work based around the new material, before beginning the language-directed tasks, will usually be of benefit to both child and therapist. This way the child has time to adjust to the new material and the therapist has time to observe this adjustment ensuring that the language-directed tasks are then provided at the level appropriate to the child.

Poor auditory–verbal processing means a total visual approach is required

Although not unsound, this approach can be severely limiting if used to exclusion. Many specialist schools dealing with speech- and language-disordered children would advocate a principally visual approach (e.g. signing or developing language through reading) because the children characteristically are poor at auditory–verbal processing (i.e. any input of language through the auditory channel). It may be necessary to begin therapy with a heavy emphasis on visual attention, performance tasks and the use of many visual cues. Eventually, however, almost all language-disordered children will have to cope with their poor auditory–verbal processing abilities and make the best possible use of them in the 'real world'. Therapy programmes should include tasks which enable the child to deal more effectively with verbal input (i.e. organising and chunking information, making use of the redundancies in language and the importance of attending to the relevant input). Once again these programmes will have to be designed in a step-wise manner in order to help the child to integrate these complex skills.

Structured language programmes are very specialised and use repetitive (and boring) equipment

There is no need to adopt an 'exclusive' approach to the treatment of language-disordered children. Most of the material that is useful for assessment and treatment can be found in any clinic. Often even better activities can be devised by using articles from the child's home or school environment. Indeed, the choice of material is really unimportant provided you know why and what you are using it for.

Some clinicians may be concerned about the number of pre-language or performance type tasks already mentioned in these sections. The use of appropriate pre-language tasks with this population cannot be emphasised enough. It is important to remember to start where the child is and, if that is pre-language (so often the case for preschool, language-disordered children), then start there. However, many clinicians will have experienced or observed a frankly boring morning when groups of children sit plodding dispiritedly through peg boards, bead threading, brick patterns and the like (the list is probably endless) and asked themselves 'Why is this going on?'. Surely if the child cannot quickly cope with an activity, then it is clearly not at the right level. The child should then be doing a different (simpler) activity or receiving adult direction (non-verbal or key words as appropriate) in order to achieve success. If not, the whole morning will have been devoted to threading two beads on a string, only reinforcing what the child cannot achieve. Ideally these tasks should be quick and rewarding so that the child is soon ready to tackle another, perhaps slightly more difficult, one. These activities do not have to be purely sedentary. Performance tasks with some physical movement can also be useful to enable the child to control distracting responses and deal with increasing environmental stimulation. Thus a non-verbal matching or sorting task, which moves on from being done at a table to including an opportunity to find things in larger space, means the child has to continue to attend to the task while coping with the distractions of the larger environment.

Treatment Ideas

Having dispensed with some popular misconceptions about styles of treatment and types of equipment or activities, we shall present some treatment ideas for this age group. Once again there is no claim for these to be particularly novel. The emphasis is on the practical and what has been effective in clinical practice over a number of years. The treatment ideas are divided into areas of difficulty (the non-starter, verbal comprehension, expressive problems) and followed by short case histories which serve to illustrate the wide range of language-disorder types and severity. These include specific examples of the treatment programmes designed for the individual children. The rest of the chapter is concerned with a discussion of the wider issues in the overall management of language-disordered children.

The non-starter

It appears to be a common ploy among overworked clinicians to abandon this group of children until they can do the kind of structured language tasks that are thought of as 'real therapy'. Whilst this may be understandable, it generally means that the family have to continue coping with the problems alone and the 'day of reckoning' is just put off for several more months. Without help, this kind of child is very seriously at risk of early educational failure and social maladjustment. Whilst time may see some spontaneous improvement, the overall cost to child and family may be considerable. It is our view that these children need early intervention. However, to begin by listing what they cannot do would take too long in most cases, and would achieve little. It would be better to begin with a question about what they can do.

These children are highly distractible with an attention span of perhaps 1−20 seconds. They are likely to present with some age-appropriate performance skills in tasks where language is not required, but on the whole these will be variable and dependent on the situation. In a highly distractible environment or a new place, it may not be possible to demonstrate these well. The children may demonstrate some basic problem-solving skills and may respond to gesture or other visual cues.

Again this will be variable and similarly situation dependent. They may have a number of negative strategies for coping with the demands of language and communication (e.g. resorting to biting, screaming or pulling to communicate). They may have no functional verbal comprehension or expression but could have inappropriate or empty social speech and very limited situational understanding. Here is an outline of the sorts of activities which have proved useful with this group.

Early attention work

As a general point, it is important to decide on a reasonable target for sustained attention. Initially, this will only be 30 seconds at the most, gradually increasing to 1 minute and then 5 minutes, and so on. However, the quality of the attention is obviously more important than the length at this stage. Suitable introductory activities include selective looking and selective listening. In a selective-looking activity, it is important to begin with a simple visual stimulus (e.g. jack-in-a-box, finger puppet). The game can be played totally non-verbally or with a few incidental key words providing these do not distract the child. The object of the game is to make the visual stimulus, which appears and disappears, sufficiently appealing to make the child want to continue looking at it or for it for the target timespan. Selective listening activities centre around listening to a sound-making object in a similar way for the target timespan. Where the child is rushing around the room, it may be necessary for the clinician to contain the child loosely within his or her arms, while presenting the stimulus activity, and then releasing the child for a short time before repeating the stimulus. The important features of this type of activity are: keep the target timespan realistic and the stimulus interesting.

The well-known 'go games' are a good example of the next stage in which listening and action are combined. Others include the use of anticipatory language in 'ready, steady, go' type games, which can often be more active (although too much activity can be destructive at this stage). Initially, the child will probably only be able to cope with one item per activity so that, for example, posting box lids may need to have some of the holes covered over so that only one is open. This will help to focus the attention and language together. Without this extra guidance, many non-starters will just continue to carry out the repetitive activity without listening. As the child progresses with the tasks it is important to build up their complexity. This may involve increasing the waiting time between selection and posting, reducing the physical restraints that are placed on the child to induce listening (the clinician can try letting go of the child now!) or increasing the number of possible items to select (either bricks to pick up or holes to put them in, but not both at once!). The important thing to remember about these transitions is that the activity must continue to be interesting and rewarding and that the child must continue to be successful. Do not move on to a more complex stage until the earlier stages have been mastered and enjoyed, not just by the child and clinician but by the child with family members and others too. Case 11 is an example of a child where this approach was used in the early stages of therapy.

Case 11

A boy was referred to speech therapy by his mother at the age of 3;9 years. He had no siblings although his mother was expecting another baby. His father was Italian, a skilled craftsman, and the mother English, not in paid employment. Only English was spoken in the home. The birth and early developmental history were unremarkable. In fact, he was described as a 'model' baby and toddler. He would play happily by himself with cars for long periods of time. He had no words by 3 years and the mother expressed her concern about this to the health visitor. She was reassured with the view that some children do talk late. Later the mother said that she had felt that some professionals had thought of her as rather overanxious about her first child.

When seen for initial assessment, he was admitted to the preschool language unit almost immediately. He had no verbal comprehension at this stage and, whilst appearing compliant, auditory attention was quite problematic. He appeared interested when language was directed to him, but this soon became a blank look and he would turn away. Symbolic play was also poor and consisted of pushing a car backwards and forwards or lining cars up repetitively. He was unable to develop new play ideas with this preferred material. He enjoyed playing with puzzles and Lego when these were demonstrated and soon succeeded at these activities. He responded well to visual demonstration and, after several weeks of intensive help, began to respond to key words, such as 'listen' and 'look'. He was silent, did not use babble or intonated vocalisation or anything resembling words. He communicated with his mother by pointing, touching her arm and making eye glides to objects. As soon as she used verbal language he was non-responsive. Initially, in the language unit, he was very withdrawn and reluctant to use his good non-verbal communication. He did make considerable progress and will be referred to again in Chapter 5.

The next stage is to move towards the integration of listening, looking, action and inhibition. In other words, the child must learn when and how to stop the activity being attended to. Once again the commands are simple words like 'go' and 'stop'. Initially physical prompts will be needed to initiate the correct response to these. Later a prefix like 'listen' or 'ready', may achieve the same result, i.e. alerting the child to attend. The aim of these activities is for the child to inhibit and control her or his behaviour at a very basic level and have fun at the same time. An action toy which the child can work may be used so that 'go' and 'stop' can be explored in a limited environment. Later the child can move on to explore the same ideas in a wider environment, e.g. having a track which the child can walk around on command. For the really adventurous, this can later be carried out in groups so that the child can also watch the way others understand the same task. By this stage, the child has begun to integrate perceptual skills and accept some adult guidance.

Early visual and performance tasks

The basic precepts of success for the child and a graded approach to introducing new aspects to the activity should continue to be followed in visual and performance tasks.

Puzzles and form boards

Language-disordered children often choose this type of activity, because they are so good at them. Once again, a time target of attention can be set for the more distractible. The child should not race through all the form boards in the clinic without having gained some tolerance of adult direction in the task. This directing may be physical or through key words. The pieces may be hidden and discovered one at a time, first on the table and later around the room.

Peg boards and bead threading

These do not need to be the dreary, repetitive tasks alluded to earlier. They can be a good way of introducing early turn-taking routines into a sedentary task so allowing child/adult cooperation to develop. The adult may initiate a simple activity, such as making a row of bricks, and then encourage the child to do the same. Once again the level of the task will vary from just putting down the same number of bricks to copying the same colour and later the same arrangement. A graded series of tasks, using the same coloured bricks to matching different coloured bricks, from the adult supplying the bricks one at a time to the child's self-selection of bricks, can all gradually be introduced providing the criteria of success by the child are adhered to. The child needs immediate feedback if he or she makes an error or if attention is lost. Do not be too quick to dismantle what has been achieved and put it back in the box. The child's success should be shared with others, most particularly the family.

Floor shapes and 'Simon Says' (non-verbal)

Once the sedentary visuospatial tasks have been mastered these skills can be transferred to action games. Clinic space may dictate the practicality of this. Where accommodation resembles a broom cupboard, the corridor may be the place for more active games (it will also give everyone else a taste of what speech therapy is and hopefully demystify it a bit). The main aims of these activities are to enable the child to cope with a more distracting environment, help him or her to imitate and initiate more complex sequences of activities and develop a sequential memory. A variety of tracks which involve shapes or feet on which the child steps, or hoops into which he or she can jump, can be used. More complicated obstacle courses are also great fun in a group situation. A non-verbal version of 'Simon Says' in which sequences of actions are directly imitated on the body can also be used. Key words like 'look' and 'ready' will be required. When errors in the sequence occur a physical prompt will help to sort out the muddle.

These basic activities should ensure that the non-starter becomes a 'starter'. The child should be attending, accepting some minimal verbal guidance and direction, listening to key words, watching for visual cues and facial expression, and beginning to inhibit and control responses, particularly errors in a positive way. Most of all the child should be aware of his or her success. These factors are illustrated in Case 12.

Case 12

This boy was referred by his health visitor at 2;10 years. His mother described him as 'a handful' and said he 'ruled the roost' at home. He would not allow any doors to be shut and never went to bed before 11 p.m. He would eat only crisps. Both parents were white-collar workers and mother worked part-time outside the home but was the major caretaker. He had two older sisters who were both healthy. The birth and early developmental history were unremarkable. He had walked early (10 months) and quickly became adventurous. He moved about rapidly and had many accidents, but could not be described as clumsy – rather as impetuous. Expressive language consisted of a continuous barrage of social phrases and questions. Listening skills were very poor; he could not listen to a short story. He would not cooperate on any formal testing and was highly distractible. Early therapy concentrated on listening skills, gaining eye contact and inhibiting empty speech. He quickly began to recognise and enjoy success so that he worked hard for verbal rewards (like 'good boy, well done', accompanied by smiles and hugs).

When attention control would allow for formal assessment (at age 3;3 years), his score on the RDLS showed a mild comprehension problem with the age-equivalent score 6 months below his chronological age (age-equivalent score 2;9 years). His understanding and use of vocabulary were so patchy that he forgot the names of even familiar household items, but talked incessantly about cartoon characters and their antics. When he did have difficulty comprehending, then expressive language became even more bizarre and inappropriate. Listening and attention work was successful in developing a greater degree of attention control (level 3 by 3;6 years). Although his eating habits did not change, he did allow doors to be closed and his bedtime routine also improved. At the age of 3;9 years he began to initiate conversation and request information with short phrases: 'We go out for play?', 'That yours, no mine, it mine!' He was willing to attempt most tasks with simple verbal direction from an adult and responded well to 'look' and 'listen'. However, he retained a rather haphazard learning style which made him a demanding member of the group.

Comprehension problems

This would seem to be the next problem requiring attention. In respect of verbal comprehension, language-disordered children will exhibit a wide range of difficulties. The level at which to start work will be determined by the assessment data. If the child presents for therapy as the 'starter' described in the last paragraph, then he or she will be attending to key words and accepting adult direction in short 'therapy' sessions. However, carry-over of this level of compliance to other situations (home, nursery) may be limited. We need to bear this in mind when suggesting appropriate language to be used with the language-disordered child in other situations. The child may have improved considerably in listening and looking behaviour, but may still need gesture and visual cues to aid comprehension. The child's attention may still be very variable, and dependent on the situation and the distractions of the environment. The seemingly very chatty child with inappropriate verbal language is easy to spot in this respect. The more inappropriate the language he or she uses the less language he or she can be assumed to have understood. Comprehension may still be partly situational and selective, such that the child attends to one aspect of the situation and ignores others. The child may exhibit islands of knowledge which appear surprising, e.g. shopping at the supermarket and being able to recognise all the brands which the family usually buys. Comprehension skills will still be abnormally affected by background noise and visual distractions, as well as any number of other unknown quantities which might be put down to the time of day, a slight cold or a change in the weather. All these can contribute to the picture of a child who finds comprehension of language quite difficult to cope with. For example, a 4-year-old, language-disordered child in a nursery class found the noisy situation in which all the other children were getting coats and going out to play quite distracting. He stood confused and alone in the middle of it. The teacher approached and presented simple language with visual cues: 'It's cold, brrr [plus gestures]. We need our ....?'. The child responded with the word 'crisps'. It is clear that at this stage the child has a very tenuous grasp of newly acquired language skills, so that these must be further consolidated and strengthened before progressing.

Visual and performance tasks

A useful way of further developing attention and comprehension is to start with what the child already knows. Familiar material with which the child has already experienced success is likely to be less daunting and distracting than new material. Many of the activities already mentioned can be further used here. Non-verbal tasks (Simple Simon) can have simple language added to them, although this must be done carefully. All the tasks can be gradually increased in complexity and distractibility so that the child's attention skills are gradually stretched. The visual memory component of the tasks can gradually be lengthened and a sequential component can be added, for example, a game called 'bricks and tubes' that requires some coloured cubes and a number of small cardboard tubes which will fit over the cubes. The adult selects a brick and puts it under a tube and the child imitates this. Both tubes are then lifted up to see if they have selected the same. For increasing complexity and a visual sequential memory component, the number of bricks and the order in which they are placed under the tubes can be gradually increased. The child has immediate feedback about errors in the sequence by direct comparison. Success is also clear and it is fun.

Most children seem to prefer to start with the abstract objects already mentioned, like bricks and beads, and move on to the real objects. Visual memory and sequencing work with objects can be done by having a matching pair of each of eight to ten different objects. The adult takes one from the array and hides it. The child has to show the matching one from his or her own array. The number of objects which the child is required to match can gradually be increased. This memory task is also influenced by other variables, such as the colour or shape of the object, which may be an important consideration if a set of small cars or animal shapes is used in which the items are very similar.

Symbolic skills

Children with comprehension problems and unstable attention control can all benefit from basic symbolic activities centred around the handling, sorting, finding and matching of everyday objects to pictures. Initially, just coping with handling everyday objects can be very distracting. This may result in the child lining things up or mechanically piling them in heaps. As a first step it may be necessary to encourage the child to group objects together in appropriate pairs – comb/brush, cup/saucer – and then use them correctly – stir cup with spoon. At first this defining of objects by their correct use will need to be done by the child in relation to him- or herself and then in relation to other people. Moving too quickly between objects will just result in the child adopting the same action for each one.

These early matching and sorting tasks do not have to be boring. As the child's attention is more controlled, a greater degree of activity can be introduced to the tasks; thus, the child can look for hidden objects around the room or sort different objects into different rooms in a doll's house. This can be extended to the home situation where the child can be encouraged to replace something in the right room.

Verbal commands

Activities which correspond to the one word level of the Derbyshire Language Scheme (Knowles and Masidlover, 1982) can be introduced at this stage. It should be possible to introduce simple verbal commands concerning everyday objects like: 'I need the sock', 'Give me the cup', 'Where's the brush'. Emphasis should be placed on the key word and a visual cue which encourages the child to scan the objects can help (like a sweep along the row of objects). This means that the child should have moved from the stage of simply echoing and looking blank or losing attention to dealing with the structured situation, attending to the stressed word and selecting the appropriate object. From this stage onwards comprehension activities which use a wide range of play and picture material can be developed.

According to the child's level of verbal comprehension, the notion of information-carrying words, as described in the Derbyshire Language Scheme (Knowles and Masidlover, 1982), can flexibly be employed in a range of play situations. We have discussed a few general principles concerning the use of the scheme in Chapter 2. Many courses are held around the country and enthusiastic clinicians are recommended to attend one of these. Ideally, language-disordered children should be able to cope with sentences containing up to four information-carrying words on entering school. Whilst this may be achieved with intensive help (this is another issue discussed later in this chapter), it is more likely that with a once, or possibly twice, weekly therapy session, coupled with a well-structured home programme and play group attendance, a more realistic goal will be the three information-carrying word level. This should provide a firm base for most classroom learning although the child will require additional support.

Whilst the three-word level of comprehension will be used for most therapy, some new work will still need to be introduced at a simpler level. This is particularly true of concept development. It is often necessary to introduce and teach concepts with a minimum of language. This may mean making initial comparisons completely non-verbal and then moving on to the key word or stressed word stage with real objects, which the child can handle, rather than pictures. Picture material can be somewhat ambiguous and sometimes there is no other way of understanding the concept than by direct experience. Thus language-disordered children will often get a better grasp of big and little by climbing into big and little boxes, and of hot and cold by tasting hot (not too hot) and cold food. It is worth while collecting objects and clear photos which illustrate many of the basic concepts (for a range of these concepts see Chapter 2), which can then be combined in a range of games. However, the following example illustrates the need to be continually vigilant in providing a wide variety of learning experiences. After 1 year of an intensive speech and language programme this child was able to sequence three actions and comprehend complex commands like: 'Put the big book on the top shelf, turn around and come to me'. However, on a visit to the park with a group of children, this skill memorably deserted her. When asked to 'Walk three steps and stand behind the tree', she stood still and pulled her dress over her head.

In order to prepare these children for classroom learning it is also important to provide opportunities for them to carry out tasks without adult direction or highly structured verbal input. This can be done with visual sequencing and classification tasks, e.g. asking the child to gather up things we can wear and then waiting and watching while he or she completes this before then going through the task alongside him or her to share the discoveries. Other tasks which could also be completed in a similar way include size ordering and sorting (getting lots of big things, putting a group of things in size order), finding things which go together, and arranging a time sequence of pictures.

Despite all this, it is clear that, whilst verbal comprehension may improve, the language-disordered child's auditory–verbal processing skills remain characteristically weak and vulnerable. They will still be having difficulty with auditory memory-based activities like a shopping game in which the child has to 'find the cornflakes, the eggs and the apples', Simon Says games where 'Simon says pat your head, rub your tummy and stamp your feet' and even longer and more complex commands like 'After you've washed your hands and cleaned your teeth go downstairs and say goodnight to daddy'. However, they can be taught to make the best use of what they have.

At the school entry stage, the child needs some strategies which will work in the classroom (and provide the teacher with the key to the strategies so that he or she can cue the child in if necessary). The first and most important thing the child has to understand confidently is not to panic if he or she is confused. This is a hard one to teach, but children who do not have this strategy are still likely to resort to echolalia or inappropriate responses. Children who have been taught from a basis of success are more likely to learn that it is alright to admit you do not understand. The easiest way of communicating that the command has not been understood is to encourage the child to ask for a repetition when this happens. This may be as simple as a gesture or sign or just the words 'again please'.

In repeating an instruction to a language-disordered child, the adult should concentrate on the key or stressed words and mark these appropriately with intonation and possibly with a visual cue like holding up a finger for each one. The child should be encouraged to shadow the message, also by using fingers if this is helpful. They can then cue themselves into action by going back to the fingers and the bits of information each one stood for. Other ways of cueing include fixing them visually in memory by remembering their position. This is possible in a game, like the shopping game, where the child can be encouraged to point to the item in the array as the command is being given. The pointing cue can then be used when the child recalls which items were requested.

Many long commands will include what might be termed 'redundant language', i.e. bits that make no difference to the child's understanding of the sentence, usually because they are obvious from the context. In the sentence: 'After you've washed your hands and cleaned your teeth, go downstairs and say goodnight to daddy please', there is a considerable amount of this redundant language. If the child is already washing his or her hands then the first part of the sentence is redundant, as presumably is daddy's location.

Clinicians can learn a great deal about the way this language is used successfully and unsuccessfully with language-disordered children by observation in various environments. Many parents are very adept at cutting all the redundancies out of language in order to ensure that the sentence remains within the child's auditory–verbal processing ability. That they do so without a formal knowledge of grammatical structures or concepts, such as 'information-carrying words', is just part of the skill required in parenting a language-disordered child.

Expressive problems

Although this section is presented separately, this is not intended to suggest that comprehension and expression cannot be worked on in parallel. Once again, a level of attention in which adult verbal guidance helps (level 3) is necessary before direct work is effective. Equally verbal comprehension such that the child can relate two pieces of information is also an important prerequisite. Even so the range of expressive language which can accompany these two factors is very wide. Some of the children will be non-verbal and some of these will be using positive strategies like gesture, pointing, pulling, intonation and facial expression to communicate. Others will still be using more negative strategies, at least occasionally, like physical force and biting or screaming. Others will be constantly jargoning, often in a quite tuneful way. However, this fairly constant stream of vocal behaviour will cut out much of the adult verbal guidance which might be provided. Others will have a small and rigid vocabulary of perhaps five words at 3 years: e.g. 'mum, dad, gimme, bye-bye'. Some will have lots of empty speech which on the surface at least may appear complex and quite sociable. However, closer inspection usually reveals that this is very repetitive and often made up of phrases gleaned from television adverts.

Signing

In the initial stages of therapy, any attempt by the child to inhibit what is not required and echo or imitate the key words provided by the adult model should be encouraged. Any non-verbal attempt to communicate effectively and appropriately should be equally rewarded. The use of a sign system may be considered in order to aid both comprehension and expression. The choice of system will depend on individual circumstances and the short- and long-term prognoses as far as learning and education are concerned. Since its introduction in the 1960s, the Paget Gorman Sign System (PGSS) has traditionally been the sign system used in many specialist schools and language units. Its advantages were discussed by Jones (1987), including the fact that it can be adapted to any level of language complexity and used alongside spoken language. Others will recommend the British Sign Language (BSL) derivatives, like the Makaton vocabulary (Walker, 1980) and Signed English. One of the advantages of the framework of the Makaton vocabulary is that it is commonly used for a wide range of children with special educational needs and is therefore more readily available as a skill among other professionals. If a BSL-based system is used, it removes the need to move the child to such a system if signing is still vital to communication at school-leaving age, when it may become an important medium of social interaction (see Chapter 6). Some will say that the young child can move from one system to another without any difficulty. However, it is easy to see that continually changing the medium of communication could have an important effect on the child's communicative confidence and self-esteem (M. Rose, personal communication).

Whatever is decided about the use of a sign system, it needs to be a joint decision adopted by the consensus of the parents and therapist, together with the agreement of the play group or nursery where necessary. Too often parents come for a second opinion assessment with fundamental questions about why another therapist has adopted a particular plan of management. Most often such questions are about the use of signing. Unilateral decisions about such things do not generally result in parental cooperation, and this may limit the child's progress. They may be suspicious about signing and see it as a social stigma. Its value must be carefully discussed, and doing this with other parents can help to alleviate some of these negative feelings. If signing is adopted, then it is important to ensure that the parents actually have an opportunity to learn the system. This does not mean leaving the attendance on a course to chance, but actively ensuring they are able to take part. We should work in partnership with parents at all stages in their child's development.

Early vocabulary for single word utterances

The single word stage will actually cover quite a range in different children, but for our language-disordered population it will mean some attempt at single units of verbal output that reliably identify different things. Some of these children will be shouting out answers along with others in their peer group. Others will be using signs with verbal labels or to cue themselves for verbal production. Some may be happy to repeat after an adult. However, the degree of intelligibility will vary and the number of words will still be limited. The question of how and in what order to teach a basic expressive vocabulary will be an important one. There are several descriptive frameworks available: PRISM L (Crystal, 1982a), Living Language (Locke, 1980), Assessment and Remediation of Concepts (Bracken, 1984); these all group areas of vocabulary together in a developmental sequence.

Alternatively, you may prefer to devise your own framework which reflects the general environment of your workplace and where the children live. It would then be possible to adapt the general framework for each child. In our case, for example, one of us works by the sea in a large town with countryside close by and the other in an inner city area by a river, but where large housing estates are common and a few small parks can be found. In both of these places, children will experience 'shopping' as a fairly regular activity. However, much will differ depending on what type of lifestyle the child's family is used to. For example, those living in bed and breakfast accommodation confined to one room will encounter a different set of concepts and vocabulary at an early age to children who live in large detached houses which contain a wide range of modern domestic technology. Early concept work in which different objects are related to separate rooms (e.g. kitchen equipment vs bathroom items) will have a different meaning to children from these very dissimilar environments. Below is a suggested basic starting point which can be readily adapted and extended.

Stage 1 vocabulary (sample)

Family members: the names and relationships like Kate, Matthew and sister, brother (and pets if relevant) etc.
Parts of the body: arms, legs, face, nose etc.
Clothes: skirt, dress, trousers, socks etc.
Favourite things: car, teddy, frog, train etc.
Room/s: door, window, furniture etc.
Meals: breakfast, dinner, lunch, tea.
Basic foods: milk, apple, bread, chips, juice etc.
Actions: washing, eating, sleeping, drinking, shopping etc.

In order to facilitate early expressive language development, it is important to focus the child onto that particular subject. This can be done in several ways:

1. Providing photos of the theme: family pictures and people doing things, favourite foods, toys, pets or things in the home, which can be looked at, matched or sorted. Essentially these need to be familiar, clear and appealing.
2. Giving the child plenty of opportunity to listen and be aware how vocabulary 'works'. In the course of a game it will be necessary to give many repetitions of the vocabulary chosen. For example: 'Let's find all the cats. Yes, that's your cat. Here's another cat. Are there any more cats?' This is fundamental before a child can be expected to produce the vocabulary him- or herself.
3. Stimulating the child to name: when the child demonstrates knowledge of the word (comprehends it) there are several ways in which the child may be encouraged to produce it. The first is the most obvious method of direct repetition. Some children will automatically move to imitation, others will need to be encouraged to imitate (for example, 'Can you say ....?', 'Now you do it' and point to child). Secondly asking a question: 'What's this?' and if necessary carrying on with other cues: 'It's a .....'. And thirdly the forced alternative: 'Is this a dog or a cat?'

All the other basic themes can be covered in the same way. Matching and sorting tasks with photos or drawings of family members or favourite toys can be used. When working on body parts, it can be fun to draw around the child's body and put the drawing on the wall. The body can be coloured in or dressed with fabric clothes. Other clothes work could include a 'jumble sale' type game where clothes can be sorted and matched. Work on meal times and daily activities could include a scrap book which could be done at home and in the clinic. None of these ideas are new and most are in fairly common use in preschool groups and clinics. The main point about using them with a language-disordered child is to limit the activities.

It is important to keep to one theme at a time, use plenty of repetition and monitor the child's progress carefully. Remember not to go beyond the child's level of comprehension in expressive tasks. Begin with tasks in which the verbal load is small, like sorting and matching. Move quickly and naturally into attempts at elicitation and praise all the child's attempts at words. Encourage signing if this seems to help initiate the word. Even if the verbal label is not forthcoming, signing should be accepted as a positive communicative response. Do not rush too quickly from one theme to the next, even if the first does not seem to be going very well. In this situation, try to think of another way of presenting the material. Here is a quick checklist which should help such an evaluation:

1. Is the child's attention level appropriate for the activity?
2. Does the child understand the concept that is being worked on?
3. Does the child know the appropriate sign (if these are used)?
4. Does the child attempt repetition?
5. Does the child respond better when this is presented in a group rather than individually?
6. Is the child enjoying the subject or activity?

For children who make slow progress with expressive language, it may be necessary to work on verbal output in the group situation. Initially this could include cause and effect games, e.g. a number of cars having a collision or building up a tower until it toppled over. Children should be encouraged to make responses like 'Oh no' and 'watch out'. Children need to remain at this level of response for some time before they are ready to attempt more direct imitation of single words.

When stuck for ideas to use with children who appear to be progressing very slowly, possible alternatives should be discussed with colleagues. There is rarely a copyright on therapy activities and two heads are often better than one. It is even better if discussed with the parents and then you can see what can be devised between you. Once there is clear evidence that the child is using the words in a range of situations, home and clinic, it is fine to move onto other themes or aspects of expressive language development.

Stage 2 vocabulary
Before introducing more vocabulary items it should be possible to begin eliciting two-word combinations (stage 2 work) from the well-used, single word vocabulary with other activities. For example, using the family photos: 'Is daddy eating? No. Is Katie eating? No. Who's eating?' To which

the child responds from the photograph 'Mummy eating–; or 'Is Nelly a fish? No. Is Nelly a dog? No. Who is Nelly?' with the response 'Nelly cat'. Forced alternatives can be used here too – 'Is it Matthew's hat or mummy's hat?' – with the response: 'Mat's hat'. At the same time it is easy to include and model negation, possession and pronouns, thus arming the child for the next stage in vocabulary development (stage 3), where many more verbs and adjectives are introduced. In these three-word phrases, the basic requirement is three elements of which the first will stand for the object, the second will be the verb and the third will stand for the subject. Objects and subjects can come from the same group. Stage three can be extended by adding attributes to the subject or object.

Stage 3 vocabulary (sample for three-word utterances)
Subjects and objects:
  People: woman, man, boy, girl, aunty, grandpa, therapist's name, siblings and peers etc.
  Park/playground: ducks, swings, trees, grass, ball, buggy etc.
  Shopping: apples, milk, nappies, beans, crisps etc.
  Television programmes: Postman Pat, Thomas the Tank Engine, Fireman Sam and others.

Verbs: walking, sitting, watching television, eating, jumping, drinking, hopping, throwing, cleaning, brushing, kicking, cuddling, clapping, pushing, drawing, painting, reading, looking, sleeping, washing, dressing, crying, laughing etc.

Attributes: big, little, up, down, in, on, under, hot, cold, old, new, open, closed, shut.

Some clinicians report an abnormality of sentence structuring such that agrammatical sentences are produced. This is also quoted as a common feature in the output of language-disordered children (Lea, 1970; Hutt, 1986). However, these examples always refer to language behaviour elicited in teaching situations and not to examples of the child's own natural language structures. For example, in a situation where the adult tries to elicit the sentence 'The man is walking' by providing the constituent elements, often with the visual support of words or symbols, the child may produce 'is walking the man' or 'walking the man is'. However, such examples do not occur in the child's spontaneous language. This type of error would appear to occur when the child is given too many words and does not have the grammatical framework on which to organise them properly. It probably indicates that more work needs to be done within simpler frames such that these are gradually built up. A scheme like the Colour Pattern Scheme (Lea, 1970) does provide one method, a colour-coded one, of representing sentence frames. The child can then place words within them in appropriate order. Case 13 illustrates a child who has a long-term problem with grammatical structure.

Case 13

This child was referred for speech therapy at the age of 3 years by her GP. He was concerned that she appeared to be unresponsive to sound although audiological examination confirmed she had normal hearing. She was the middle child of three girls. The other two were developing normally, and there was no family history of speech and language problems. Her birth and early developmental history were unremarkable. At the initial meeting, she cooperated well with formal assessment. At a chronological age of 3;0 years, she scored an age equivalent of 2;9 years on the RDLS. She was untestable on the expressive scale. She was admitted to a language unit at the age of 3;3 years. After the first 6 months it was apparent that her comprehension skills were progressing very slowly. Reassessment on the RDLS at a chronological age of 3;9 years gave an age-equivalent score of 3 years for verbal comprehension and 1 year for expressive language. Her expressive language consisted of single nouns in lists with gaps in between each one in which she would hold her breath or insert a short vowel. The effect was to produce a non-fluent language style in which meaning was difficult to discern out of context. For example, a description of an outing to the park sounded like this: 'Mummy /ə/ me /ə/ Katie /ə/ Elsie [the dog] /ə/ [breath] /ə/ go /ə/ walk /ə/ flowers. This was interpreted to mean 'Mummy, me, Katie and Elsie went for a walk and saw some flowers? This pattern of expressive language continued. At a chronological age of 5 years her verbal comprehension of the RDLS was 3;9 years and expressive language was 2;3 years. An extended example of her language is given here (A = adult and C = child, discussing a picture sequence):

A: Here we are, let's look at this one shall we?
C: OK.
A: What can you see here (pointing)?
C: A man.
A: Yes, what's he doing?
C: Drive a .... drive a ..... car.
A: It's not a car is it? Look. What's that on the back [pointing]?
C: Milk! He drive the milk!
A: Yes that's right, milk. Milk bottles. So who's this man?
C: A milk ..... a man.
A: Where's he going here [pointing]?

     C: He go up a gate. He go up there [points at path]. He go to
        door.

     A: Now what's happening?

     C: He put the milk . . . . . he go to . . . he go up . . . . the end!

     A: OK. Just tell me the story. Is it morning or night?

     C: Don't know.

     A: When do you get your milk?

     C: In the house . . . . . my drink.

     A: Do you like milk?

     C: Yes!

This child demonstrates several levels of difficulty, including comprehension. Expressive language was non-fluent, telegrammatic and there was evidence of perseveration in the use of some responses and sentence structures. Although her age-equivalent level was recorded as 2 years at this stage, the above sample is clearly not characteristic of the expressive language of a normally developing 2 year old.

Once the child has achieved stage 2 it is usually much easier to achieve an immediate response or repetition in stage 3 of expressive language development. The syntactic ability to combine object, verb and subject into these S-V-O type sentences will often enable the child to make considerable self-initiated progress through their own discoveries. It is therefore worth spending extra time on this and engaging in a lot of reordering of the possible elements in order to demonstrate this capacity to the child. It is this reordering that is an essential skill in creativity with language.

It is well worth exploring different ways of including expressive language development tasks in a variety of situations, including manipulating real-life events. For example, if the usual order of a set of activities is changed, the child will have an opportunity to express this to the adult. This can only be done successfully when it will not cause severe anxiety or behavioural disturbance within the group, but it can be a way of eliciting expressive language. Instead of the usual milk at break time, an apple or orange could be presented, or play time could be changed for story time or rest time.

The use of humour or incongruity can also elicit expressive language at this stage, particularly those involving why, because, negation, questions, inversion, plurals and pronouns. From a set of incongruous pictures children may produce sentences like: 'Why he got that hat?', 'She not got one . . . . a nose', 'He can't get out . . . . that stuck'. Role-playing has already been discussed as a strategy for earlier stages of expressive language work. By this stage the child should be able to cope with the idea of role reversal such that he or she is able to take the adult's part in the game. This allows the child to gain an understanding of the perspective of others, as well as using language structures for directing others.

Stage 4 vocabulary

At the fourth stage of expressive language development, a larger range of vocabulary is incorporated into increasingly complex utterances. Importantly, for the first time some vocabulary begins to extend beyond the child's direct experience. However, it is still important to base this new information on what the child already knows. A good way of doing this is to work on themes which involve collections of objects and planned outings with family and staff. In this way vocabulary collections about animals, transport, clothes, shops etc. can be extended together with appropriate verbs and concepts. Important social events can become theme focuses: Christmas, bonfire night, holidays. The Derbyshire Language Scheme (Knowles and Masidlover, 1982) also provides a number of suggestions for a gradual approach to the development of sentence structure.

The Language-disordered Child's Knowledge of Phonology and Prosody

The speech of language-impaired children may contain evidence of difficulty at the phonological or prosodic level. In such cases it may be described as unintelligible or indistinct. The development of speech–sound contrasts (phonology) may be delayed or deviant. Some language-disordered children's language development reflects a disorder at the phonological level (see Chapter 1). The child's knowledge of the rhythmic components of words, the stress, syllable structure and intonation may be impaired (prosody), and this may be reflected in a flat and monotonous style of delivery in which word boundaries are unclear. Activities which concentrate on these levels of language should be incorporated into a language programme as appropriate. They are a useful precursor to direct work on speech–sound contrasts which should help the child to manipulate and internalise phonological information more effectively. This has been found to have a beneficial effect on the child's ability to progress with early reading skills (Thompson, 1984).

Rhythm work

Language-disordered chaildren have been shown to demonstrate deficiencies in their development of rhythm (Lea, 1980). In a programme aimed at developing such skills, a hierarchical approach is to be preferred. It must be remembered that the child needs to experience success at each stage. A start is made with a demonstration of the rhythm of the child's own name and the names of others: 'Matthew' has two beats and 'Samantha' has three; then the move is on to include the rhythmic pattern of the names of common objects: 'table' has two beats and 'potato' has three. Following this work is towards an understanding of this concept in multisyllabic words which contain different patterns: 'crocodile' has three beats with the emphasis on the first and third, whilst 'banana' also has three but the emphasis is on the middle one. A drum could be used to demonstrate the differences in the amount of stress on each syllable.

Pitch work

This is started by establishing the difference between high and low pitch using a xylophone or chime bars, and then the concept of medium tones between these two extremes is added. The child should be encouraged to imitate a simple pattern of two tones using the visual cue available from watching the adult model. Later a move is made towards the child copying the pattern from sound alone. When a vocal component is added to the pattern initially, make sure it is non verbal. For example, the child copies the adult model in which the sound 'ah' is added as a glide over the two-tone model of one high and one low pitched note. This is developed further by adding animal noises over the pitch changes like 'hee-haw' and 'quack-quack'. From here it is possible to move on to simple stereotyped phrases within the child's repertoire, such as 'OK', 'alright', 'bye bye' and later to longer and more complex phrases in a step-wise progression.

The characteristics of sounds

Most children who present with disordered phonology as a part of their language problem still have a sound system that is rule governed, systematic and predictable. Dean and Howell (1985) infer from this that the child's problem is at the processing rather than the articulatory level. They go on to suggest that the way to develop the child's sound system is to give them first an awareness of that system and also the level of communicative effectiveness which results when it is used. This is called a metaphon approach to phonology therapy. Metaphon refers to the way in which this approach allows the child to develop a linguistic awareness of the sounds themselves, their properties and how they are used. In the first stage, this means making the properties of the phonemes more opaque and, in the second stage, providing feedback about how effective communication has been. By these methods the child will then, according to the piagetian framework which this theory adopts, change the sound system in order to make communication more effective. In practice this means a two-phase therapy programme.

Phase 1

In order to make the phonemes more opaque, labels need to be attached to them which describe their characteristics. The child may be asked to describe the phonemes him- or herself. Two major groups of characteristics need to be agreed on: manner and place of articulation. The characteristics of manner which can form a starting point are voicing (described as loud or soft) and stopping (described as short or long). Articulatory placement of the phonemes within the oral cavity can be used as a visual cue for the children. These can be colour coded: red for bilabials, blue for alveolars, yellow for velars. Initial exercises will need to ensure that the concepts of size, length and colour used are well known to the child. The child's task is to discriminate, both auditorily and visually, which of the sounds is being produced in the adult model.

Phase 2

In this phase the aim is to give the child an awareness of the extent to which his or her own system matches the adult model. The child receives feedback about how clearly he or she was understood. This work can be done in any popular game in which the child is motivated to produce words and essentially involves the child producing a distinction between minimal pairs of words (e.g. 'tea' and 'key' or 'goat' and 'coat'). The listener has to decide how well he or she has understood what the child said and feed back as appropriate. The properties of the sound established in phase 1 can be used here as a cue to help identify which sound was intended when communication breaks down.

The kinds of activities which can be incorporated are wide. The programme should be well structured and include activities at the non-speech sound level initially, working through the phoneme and word level. These are well discussed by Dean and Howell (1986). A programme developed for an individual child is described by Jarvis (1989). She considers the questions of what to teach, how long for and by what method, and describes how each of the phonological processes is worked on in turn. Clinical experience using this system with phonologically impaired children suggests it can be done successfully in a group of 4 year olds, which is small (up to four or five children) by two therapists working together (one modelling and one helping the children to monitor what is happening) and working intensively (every day for 3 hours a week). The advantage of the system is that it is based on success and even the most reluctant children have enjoyed it. The activities can be fun and the children enjoy helping each other make their communication more effective.

There is no reason why all this work should be individual and static. Providing the child's attention control is at a suitable level, then group activities and those which contain movement (particularly good for rhythm work) can be included. The child's need for good attention control cannot be emphasised enough in this work, because it is fundamental to further progress in auditory processing skills.

Case 14 illustrates a child who had a tendency to use an unstressed short vowel to link syntactic elements.

Case 14

This boy (aged 4 years) was referred for speech therapy by his mother. She had become concerned that he was due to start school in a further 6 months and was not yet speaking. However, he was a good communicator, using a combination of mime, gesture, grunting and facial expression. By this means he was able to convey quite complex sequences, providing the context was known. On his first visit to the clinic he described a trip to see his uncle the previous day; he went on a train (gesture and mime), played darts (mime) and his uncle hurt his arm (gesture and mime). His older brother had attended speech therapy for a mild degree of language delay at the age of 4, and the problem was resolved by the age of 5 years.

Initial assessment of verbal comprehension was age appropriate (an age equivalent of 4;3 years at a chronological age of 4;0 years on the RDLS). Expressive verbal skills could not be tested. He responded well to a structured programme of eliciting language from single words to two-word combinations and quickly progressed to the subject–verb–object stage. At the age of 4;6 years, he used a process of substituting an unstressed short vowel (the schwa) for omitted unstressed grammatical elements at the sentence and word level which finally disappeared 9 months later.

For example:

Target	Response
The boy is climbing the ladder.	The boy /ə/ climb /ə/ ladder.
Mummy's going to the shops.	Mummy go /ə/ shops.
That one's mine	That /ə/ mine.
My dad's got a new car.	My dad /ə/ new car.

This feature is fairly common in the language-disordered population, because such individuals try to cope with increasing syntactic complexity (Leonard, 1979). The boy's entry into mainstream school was delayed for half a term, and he began for afternoons only at 5 years of age. Both teachers and speech therapists agreed that he settled in well. At the end of the first term a new member of staff, learning that he had local speech therapy, reported that his only outstanding problem was a difficulty in the articulation of /kr/ clusters.

The Use of Language and Communication Skills

The aim for all language-disordered children must be for them to become confident, if not totally competent, language users. Structured language work will be important in this, but it will not teach them everything they need to know about using language in everyday life. Young language-disordered children can gain much confidence from using their new-found skills in their everyday situation, but they will probably need help to do this. Generalisation of skill will not usually take place automatically. It may be necessary to focus on particular areas of pragmatic ability one at a time, as the programme progresses, to ensure that the child does learn how to use the language skills that therapy has been teaching. This is to be preferred to leaving pragmatic abilities until the end of the child's time in therapy as a kind of afterthought.

It is important to remember that not all pragmatic abilities are verbal. The non-verbal ones have an important place and may be easier for the young language-impaired child to use, at least initially. A gesture of greeting, facial expression or eye glide as a response during conversation may be an appropriate first stage. From here simple single words and phrases can be used appropriately in communicative exchanges in pretend play, role-play and real-life conversations, particularly at home. The child can be given the opportunity to direct the adult, or another child, and thereby gain experience of the power of effective communication. Some possible activities include:

1. Going around an obstacle course: giving instructions can be done with just a few words and other performatives, like 'careful' and 'watch out', can also be used as appropriate.
2. A large floormat, road layout with cars: again a few words can be used to direct the scene within a simple exchange. An unexpected situation can be included, like an accident, in order to help the child plan the use of new language, rather than just what has been rehearsed. Remember that non-verbal signals to warn or indicate change are also acceptable ways of communicating.
3. Setting up an everyday situation which can have a number of possibilities: it may be necessary to have other adults take part in some

of these, or perhaps some children who do not have language disorders, so that the child and therapist can see what happens. Picture card sequence can also be used but they are rarely as exciting as real action. Begin with the simple everyday things like an exchange over breakfast. The child asks for milk and is given a banana. Now what should he or she do? Once again, remember that non-verbal skills may be used here. The situation can then be acted out again, at first with the same outcome, so that the child can respond as discussed. Later, a whole range of different outcomes can be introduced.

Wider Management Issues

So far we have discussed a range of typical difficulties encountered in preschool, language-disordered children and presented some ways in which to deal with these within a treatment programme. Now we aim to set this information within the context of the how, when and where this treatment takes place and with whom. Whilst professionals will vary on the types of provision they advocate for any one language-disordered child, the aim must always be to provide a clearly structured treatment programme which will be responsive and specific to each child. Above all, consistency and continuity must be a fundamental part of this aim. Unfortunately, however, recent trends seem to suggest that too often decisions about the needs of language-impaired children are made on the basis of local or national politics which dictate financial provision and the availability of staff and resources. Within these often frustrating constraints the professional still aims to provide the best service for each child. The following issues are important factors to consider in service provision.

Parental involvement

Working with young language-disordered children within the home and tackling problems at source is certainly desirable (Stevenson, Bax and Stevenson, 1982). However, it should not be considered an easy option in terms of the adequate provision of speech therapy for this group. Designing and implementing a home programme takes a good deal of time and energy on the part of the therapist. The ongoing evaluation of such a programme will involve further time and also discussion with the parents. Whilst it may be possible to utilise a common skeleton or outline for most programmes with young language-disordered children, all will require considerable development and child-specific additions to be really effective. A home programme may sound like a good idea, but it can result in considerable additional pressure being put on home life which may already be quite hectic. This factor will need to be considered and discussed sensitively.

The benefits parents can gain by working through a treatment programme can be considerable. They may begin to see the scope of the child's difficulties more clearly, thus enabling them to add their observations to assessment and discussion about the child with greater confidence and clarity. As they become more informed about the problem, they can also see the child's strengths more clearly and encourage these in the course of family life. However, it is important to remember that their major role is as the child's parents and not just a spare-time therapist; the child needs them to be parents and not necessarily have the whole family engaging in language-related activities all the time. Full and active parental involvement at any time may not be possible for a variety of reasons. These may be related to real or perceived difficulties in other aspects of personal and family life, including financial, social, psychological, health or intellectual factors. Equally the child may not find it easy to accept guidance from the parents and other help may need to be sought in this respect (e.g. from health visitor, child guidance clinic, social worker etc.). Where parental involvement is limited other possible considerations which might be considered include:

1. A friend, relative, neighbour, older step-sibling or local volunteer may become a partner in the home programme. When considering this option it is important to understand the relationship this person has and will have with the family.
2. Practical help may be sought from other agencies. The possibility of providing a programme for the family at a family centre or through a family aide with the help of social services or the voluntary sector may be considered.
3. Involvement by play group or nursery staff working with the child. The child may have been placed in a nursery or play group for part of the day or week. It may be an appropriate part of their work to carry out language-based activities in partnership with the therapist. This may depend on the amount of time they have available and some additional training input.

Depending on how effective these options are, and the severity of the problem, it may be necessary to consider a more radical course which would include more intensive help for the child.

Intensive therapy

An assessment centre or language unit where the child attends for 3–5 half-day or whole-day sessions a week for a block of 6–10 weeks will provide more intensive help for the severely impaired child. In such a setting, speech therapists, teachers, nursery nurses, parents and others can work together with the child and also actively support the home programme as necessary. However, personal experience suggests that the provision of such resources is decreasing rather than increasing. This may be due, in some part, to financial constraints but conflicting research evidence and philosophies also play a part. The idea that work with language-impaired children should start as soon as possible has gradually developed over the last 10 years and it seemed, initially at least, as if research findings support this view (Clezy, 1978; Cooper, Moodley and Reynell, 1978; Ward and Kellett, 1982; Schiefelbusch and Pikar, 1986).

Recently there has been a change in this trend towards early intensive provision for language-disordered children. Follow-up studies which have considered the effectiveness of speech and language units (Turner and Vincent, 1987) seemed to indicate that intensive therapy was not significantly related to eventual outcome. A closer look at these studies in language units which were educationally based, reveals that the youngest children at entry were 3;6 years old (mean age of 6 years). Perhaps these findings merely reflect the need to admit younger children. A follow-up study of 3–5 year olds who attended a preschool language unit (Urwin, Cook and Kelly, 1988), seen again at a mean age of 8;3 years, showed that 84% of them were in mainstream education and making progress with little or no additional support. A longitudinal study of language and motor development in 4–5 years olds (Bishop and Edmundson, 1987) considered the variability of the therapy which the children had received to be too great to include it as a predictor of outcome.

The overall effect of this wealth of research seems to be the development of a 'wait and see' approach to the provision of intensive therapy for language-disordered children. Unfortunately, this may well mean that a language-disordered child has to fail in mainstream education before an appropriate special needs provision is made. It is to be hoped that this philosophy proves to be transient. The child who experiences continued failure learns much that is negative about self-esteem and confidence. It may be that the therapist has to consider other ways of providing more intensive help for preschool, language-disordered children. A number of questions may be the starting point for such a discussion (these will be considered further in Chapter 7):

1. What resources are required to run a small language group two or three times weekly? This needs to include staffing, space and equipment.
2. Are there enough children of this age in the district/clinic area who need this provision?
3. Are these children similar or very different in the type(s) of language problems they have? It is important to consider the homogeneous or heterogeneous nature of the group when considering the number of children who could be included and the number of staff needed.
4. Is the need sufficient to warrant a re-scheduling of other clinical commitments? If more staff are not available, it may be necessary to

consider the ways in which present availability to staff can be used to greater effect.

5. Will this plan fit with the policies of the district service? The way the service is organised will vary from district to district and depend on the management styles which those who lead the service exercise. Some will respond more favourably to a 'grass roots' initiative than others.

6. Could other people or agencies be involved? The parents may be considered able to take a more active role in running the group in partnership with the therapist(s). Others, including health visitors or volunteers, may also be considered as possible partners.

Sharing information and training co-workers

An ideal situation might be one in which the parents and all other co-workers are fully aware of the scope of language disorder, and what it means in practical terms and particularly with regard to the future development of communication skills and future learning. Obviously, in practice this is not fully possible. Parents may gain a thorough understanding of their child's problems, but find it difficult to develop a general overview. Support and discussion groups may prove a useful focus in which to exchange views and information. It is however, inevitable that parents' views of language disorder will remain highly individual and dependent on their own experiences. Similarly related professionals and other co-workers will also be influenced by previous experience and training. They may work from a particular view of language disorder, perhaps seeing it as one specific syndrome with a set of attached clinical features; they may continue to work within a definition by exclusion rather than taking a wider and more inclusive view. Others may see the problem as a part of a general or overall learning difficulty and, whilst they may observe the symptoms, fail to see them as connected. Some will see the problem as essentially an emotional or behavioural one.

Encouraging a group of professionals to share a common vision and gain from the views of others is not always possible. However, when working in the field of childhood disability in general and language disorder in particular, experience suggests that, whilst it is demanding, it can be achieved within a multidisciplinary team. Learning from the experiences of others requires a commitment to work with them both clinically and non-clinically. This will mean clinical work being carried out in close proximity (as discussed in Chapter 3) and time for administrative planning and sharing of new information recognised as essential parts of the team's activities. Meetings will need to be well coordinated with a clear focus and opportunities for evaluating the team's goals. Time for the people to share new information also needs careful planning so that everyone's needs may be considered and contributions made, as appropriate, by the range of people involved. Learning about language disorder does not just involve a number of sessions of someone telling the rest what he or she thinks they need to know. Ways of deepening a joint understanding of language disorder will be further discussed in Chapter 7.

Let us return to the essential clinician's checklist proposed by Coombes (1987). We have discussed the what to do and how to do it, and even made some points about where, but have not yet considered when to start and when to stop, which will now be discussed.

When to start

The usual starting time for the assessment and treatment process is around 3 years of age. The child is usually referred as the result of having failed to pass a developmental screening check at a local clinic, or by a GP responding to a parental request. However, children do present at a younger age, which is to be encouraged. This may be because they already fall into an at-risk group, perhaps because they present with a syndrome in which speech and language difficulties are of common occurrence such as cleft palate (see Appendix I for further syndromes associated with speech and language difficulties). Some districts do operate a screening policy at a younger age, which identifies children at 2 years of age as having potential difficulty in speech and language development. There would appear to be no standard procedure in use in the UK for the identification of children with language disorder.

Clinical experience and research literature continue to confirm that children present for initial assessment after the age of 5 years with little evidence of previous contact with speech therapy services (Kellett and Ward, 1980) or a clear idea of their speech and language needs (Martin, 1984). There may be many reasons for later referral:

1. Language disorder may not be recognised as a reason for deviant development in that locality (health district or education authority).
2. Resources within the locality may be limited to certain groups and certain ages so that young language-disordered children do not receive specific help.
3. The child's language disorder may not have been recognised by the local professionals due to inexperience.
4. The waiting list system in operation may mean that, although the child was referred earlier, it has taken perhaps 2 years for him or her to reach the top of the list and therefore be seen.
5. The problem has been recognised, but insufficient clinical time has meant that intensive help has not been possible.
6. The parents' anxieties have been dismissed as a result of various

well-intentioned people prejudging the situation in some way. The parents may be unaware that they can make a direct referral.
7. The child has 'slipped through the net' for any number of reasons.

The degree to which any one therapist can make a constructive contribution to removing these reasons for late referral will vary. Where they are bound up with the overall management structure of the service it may be more difficult and personally demanding. A full knowledge of the system, and clear information concerning the clinical situation (statistics etc.), as well as recent research evidence, will be required when planning to present an alternative strategy to remove some of these reasons from the list. Some may just require more efficient local publicity.

Those who work with preschool children usually consider the age of around 3 years as an excellent time to begin play group or nursery. In a child who is developing normally, motor, social and communication skills are maturing rapidly and he or she is becoming more self-reliant. Practical factors, such as an ability to accept separation from parents, independent toileting and eating and drinking skills, as well as an ability to accept adult verbal guidance, listen to group instructions and the development of creative play ideas, are all important when considering whether a child is able to join a particular group. The phrase often used to evaluate this is: 'Is the child ready?' or 'When the child is ready'. Some speech therapists also use this criterion when considering children suitable for therapeutic intervention. However, 3-year-old language-disordered children are such a heterogeneous group that, if this was always the method adopted to determine when to begin, then it would mean that some children would never get started.

The child who presents with specific expressive problems often performs age appropriately in all other areas of development, but many other language-disordered children will be operating at a lower level in some aspects of social and motor skills. For children with severe attention problems and possibly accompanying behavioural problems, intervention can usefully begin between 2 and 2;6 years. Working with parents and children through a home programme can be very effective for listening, attention and early communication skills. The preschool child may already have learned a great deal about failure to communicate and this could already have resulted in low self-esteem (Clezy, 1978). It is possible to begin by modelling more appropriate social and interactional skills – developing looking and awareness of others, gaining attention and taking turns at a very basic level (Schiefelbusch and Pikar, 1986), which can have very positive effects for the child and family. The result can be a general lessening of anxieties and family dynamics and interactions return to a more normal pattern (Clezy, 1978; McDade, 1981).

When to stop

The manner in which this question arises will depend on the view of language disorder taken by the clinician. Many will prefer to describe the child as 'severely delayed', suggesting a view that the child will eventually catch up, perhaps because they consider the term 'disorder' to be too medical or synonymous with a poor prognosis. For us, the term 'disorder' is a description of one type of uncommon developmental pattern which can, if not recognised and remediated effectively, lead to severe and persistent difficulties which limit a child's overall potential. As the population of language-disordered children is so heterogeneous, then some will initially present with very severe problems and make considerable progress, so that their problems resolve. Others will have greater long-term difficulties which, whilst they make progress, will persist beyond the preschool years.

It is unlikely that a preschool language-disordered child would be completely discharged from therapy by school age. It is possible that he or she will have made significant progress so that only periodic review, occasional discussion with parents and school staff or perhaps some intervention during school holidays will be required. Children who do still require regular therapy should not continue to work on unrewarding and unevaluated language programmes for months on end. This is demoralising for the child, family and therapist. Therapy should be considered in blocks, each block being thought of as the time required to achieve a particular and relevant goal. Blocks of 5–10 weeks might be appropriate depending on the goal set and the intensity of the therapy. There will be some children who require continued intervention after the age of 5 years, and it is their needs which will be discussed in the next chapter.

Chapter 5
Treatment and Management of School-aged Children with Language Disorders

Summary

This chapter seeks to address the problems of language-impaired children within mainstream education. The management of local clinical resources is discussed with a view to meeting the needs of the children and their class teachers. The development of specialist units and classes, their selection criteria and the case for early intervention are issues considered as part of the current debate.

Introduction

The reception class teacher said the following:

> Will the paint people stop what they're doing, put their paintings on the radiator to dry, clean their brushes and hands and sit down at the piano. Will the sand people stop what they're doing, take off their aprons and sit down by the piano. Will the measuring people tidy away all the counters and sit at the piano. Will the people making papier-mâché models for their mummies put them to dry and tidy away all the paper; then sit down by the piano. We're all going to have some songs.

This memorable speech welcomed a language-disorderd child (see Case 11) to his first experience of mainstream education. Indeed, this could be a typical example of an instruction given in many group situations in mainstream schools, and it demonstrates just how difficult it is to prepare a language-disordered child for integration. The child, to his credit, realised he was a 'sand person' and appeared to concentrate hard on the instructions directed to his group. He started to undo his apron. However, the 'measuring people' and 'papier-mâché people' intervened and he began to look confused. Therapy with this boy had included considerable work on this type of situation and it was pleasing to see what happened next. He did not panic. He looked round at the other 'sand people' and carefully followed them to the piano, glancing at the teacher regularly to check this was the right thing to do. He was able to demonstrate that the strategies he had been taught did work.

Whilst such language-disordered children's problems are concentrated in language skills, all learning involves language to some extent. Thus the child's difficulties become more diffuse, involving abstract concepts, manipulation of vocabulary as well as poor auditory memory. Most important of all is the child's ability to pay attention to what is directed to her or him and disregard the rest; to be able, in a sense, to filter the relevant information for her- or himself. Such a skill will involve learning from peers and adults as well.

The ideal provision for children with severe speech and language disorders should meet the following criteria:

1. It should begin early.
2. It should be intensive.
3. It should be specific to the child's needs.
4. It should be structured rather than just involving general language stimulation principles.
5. It should be consistent.
6. It should be built on the child's success.

However, 'such provision has tended to develop on an ad hoc basis, with little evidence of any consensus about who needs it or how it is best delivered' (Pocklington and Hegarty, 1982). We wonder whether, at the beginning of the 1990s, it is possible to say that this statement no longer applies. There clearly are some unresolved problems relating to the rapid increase in the number of language units and the staff working in them. Working practices have of necessity, developed via an approach that might be termed 'learn while you work together', and individual experiences are shared through training and group meetings. This has gradually lead to a developing consensus on how to deliver services to language-disordered children, although what any one language unit offers will depend to some extent on the experience of the staff and how much access they have to the material and information available. The development of an effective curriculum will also be dependent on the working relationship between staff and families and their understanding of teamwork.

One of the most difficult issues for language unit staff remains the admission policy (Pocklington and Hegarty, 1982). The criteria for admission may be set or rather arbitrary; keeping to a strict policy or waving the rules can both have advantages or disadvantages. Greater flexibility in a positive sense can ensure that children with general as well as specific language and learning problems receive a thorough and ongoing assessment of language strengths and needs before being referred to a more appropriate long-term placement. Unfortunately, due to the limited number of places in most units, it can sometimes result in a number of admissions which then reduce the availability of places for other urgent cases. The following sequence of events illustrates this point.

A language unit, catering for children aged 3–7 years and attached to a first school, had three vacancies. There were three children under 4 years of age with severe language problems, who were due to be admitted and who had already visited the unit with their families prior to a starting date being arranged. Then, in quick succession, three other admissions had to take priority so that the original three were not able to take up the places. First, a 6-year-old girl already in the unit, and due to move on, could not do so. This was because the school which was to receive her could not get the promised provision of an infant welfare assistant she was thought to need. The second vacancy was taken by a 6;6-year-old boy with severe language and behavioural problems. He had been offered a place the previous year, but family and teachers had agreed that he should stay in mainstream school for a further period. However, a rapid deterioration in his behaviour had resulted in a crisis admission, since it was not proving possible to contain him in school. Finally, a family moved in from another district with a sheaf of reports and recommendations which indicated unit placement for the child, now also over 6 years old. Thus the three preschool children had to wait at least another year for placement, by which time they were nearly school age.

In summary then, language unit staff may have little or no say in who is ultimately admitted. Where they can be directly involved they are in a better position to identify which children can best be helped (Pocklington and Hegarty, 1982). Obviously children may arrive late in the unit because of earlier 'blocks' in the system, when other children are prevented from moving on. If this is the case, staff may have a relatively short time to try and work with the complex problems before the child is too old for that unit. Children may be placed in a language unit for other reasons, but not principally because of their language problem. The successful integration and return of the child to mainstream school can also be problematic. Ways in which language-disordered children can be helped to manage better in mainstream education will be discussed later in this chapter. It is important to remember, of course, that some severely language-disordered children will not return to mainstream school and will require long-term special provision.

The help which a language-disordered child receives in mainstream school does not, unfortunately, always reflect his or her specific needs. A number of factors will influence this provision.

Early identification

It is highly likely that a child with severe language problems is already known to speech therapists by school age. If so, there will be notes and reports which describe the child's development over time and outline strengths and weaknesses. Early evidence of language disorder should be shared with health visitors, medical officers and educational psychologists. What happens to the child depends very much on good liaison between services at both departmental and personal levels. Meetings between these services, where the progress of preschool and school-aged children can be regularly discussed and monitored, often provides better information than a formal written report alone. Presenting a case verbally may provide a useful way of sharing information and knowledge regarding the scope of language disorder and its probable effects on classroom learning. As always, setting up and maintaining these communication links is dependent upon the individual participants, their commitment and enthusiasm and, most importantly, their time limitations. Early identification of the problem is vital, because it may lead to a statement of educational need according to the provision of the 1981 Education Act. At the very least it will begin to quantify the particular areas of need within a district/area so that the possibility of setting up language unit/class(es) is discussed as a part of future policy. This does not rule out the need for practical suggestions for working with language-disordered children in mainstream school with or without additional support, which this chapter seeks to address.

Problems of assessment

When considering a language-disordered child's educational needs the following attitude may be encountered among some clinicians:

> Referring a child to another professional or for a second opinion and waiting for the report can be disappointing. At best it may confirm what you already know and at worse it provides a limited or distorted view of the child's abilities.

We need to consider what underlies this type of view of the assessment procedure. It must be remembered that not even the most ingenious professional can assess a child in a vacuum. If the professional concerned has only limited background information and a short time to complete the assessment, he or she is likely to use a formal assessment which will provide an age-equivalent or standard score. The results may simply reflect how well or how poorly the child performed within that test situation on that particular day. It may be that the referring person only receives from the referral as much as he or she is prepared to contribute. This is why it is really worth meeting and discussing individual children with other professionals on a regular basis; it usually generates a number of positive effects. A more complete picture of the range, severity and variety of language problems within the district/area is established. These may then be identified earlier, which in turn can lead to the development of improved services. A combined approach to the assessment of children with language disorder may develop from close liaison with the school where the child is finally placed.

Identifying problems in the classroom

However often a therapist visits a school to discuss individual children, he or she may still find that the ideas provided for language work within the classroom are not taken up. This is not really surprising when considering that in order to carry out a language programme, a teacher must first, correctly identify the variety of problems associated with language disorder, then focus on the child's specific needs in that context and finally set about working on these effectively in the classroom. The class teacher's expertise is not in speech and language but in education of children, the development of a curriculum for individuals and groups, and the planning and presentation of the material which makes up that curriculum. The teacher is concerned with providing an interesting and enjoyable learning experience for the child which will enable the child to achieve his or her potential. The teacher may be very accurate in the general assessment of the problem, for example, the child does not listen, the child's speech is unclear, the child will not carry on with any activity alone, the child always chooses to play with bricks or in the 'home corner'. The speech therapist, however, has been trained to make a differential diagnosis from these general observations which tune him or her into the child's language problem for the purpose of planning intervention. Thus, given that the child does not listen, the speech therapist would wish to consider possible contributing factors, for example, a low level of attention, a possible hearing problem, the complexity of the instructions, the complexity of the task and so on. It is clear that teachers and speech therapists working together can make formidable teams. However, teamwork and liaison within the classroom are not without their own problems.

Liaison within the classroom

When identifying problems children have within the classroom situation, some may be more easily identified than others, for example, physical difficulties, general learning problems, and social, behavioural, visual and hearing problems. Perhaps this is because of the complex way in which symptoms and causes interact in the language-disordered group. Thus, when the traditional definition by exclusion is used they appear as a remnant which is poorly described. The child may present as if he or she does not hear, has a learning problem, seems immature, or received limited opportunities as a preschool child. It is therefore quite likely that the teacher may perceive and group such children quite differently from the speech therapist (Urwin, Cook and Kelly, 1988).

The speech therapist should have a full and sympathetic knowledge of the classroom situation, and the skills and resources that are required to teach within it. The situation may mean that a language programme which works well within the clinic cannot be implemented in the classroom for practical reasons; lack of individual staff time is probably the most significant one. The classroom environment, in its widest sense, and its effect on learning must be considered. Some aspects of the child's language problem may become more apparent at school, rather than in the clinic. Such new variables as the distraction of the peer group, background noise and distracting material, may adversely affect the child's performance. It is important to remember that the majority of children can learn in this way.

Watching the way the other children and teachers interact can further highlight the deficiencies of the language-disordered child. Watching a teacher work with 20–30 reception-class children for a morning can be an eye opener. For the newcomer and observer, the general noise and activity level may appear such that it is hard to discern the underlying structure of the session or discuss long-term plans with the teacher, or give specific ideas and examples of what to do about particular language problems within the themes being worked on that term. Several visits may be necessary to familiarise oneself with the routine and investigate the possibilities, before the teacher and therapist can plan and implement ideas together.

Monitoring progress within the classroom

Language-disordered children can be identified and dealt with appropriately within the classroom but additional support, in the form of individual or small group work, may be required. Such a decision or plans for the child's future needs will have to consider other factors, such as the child's personality, family support and the school's ability to manage the problem long term. For the language-disordered child in mainstream school, it is essential that her or his strengths and weaknesses are fully understood and progress evaluated regularly by the people involved. It may be that the teacher and speech therapist identify an area of language work which cannot be tackled in a large group, or perhaps a general pattern of failure is recorded where the child is slipping further and further behind peers. It is important that the educational psychologist, as the person responsible at present for the assessment of the child's educational needs, is kept fully informed about the progress the child makes within the current provision. Although, as schools take on their own budgets, it may be that the services of educational psychologists are used differently. Schools could choose to bring in a wide range of professional expertise and assessments will no longer be the educational psychologist's domain alone. Identifying and documenting any serious shortfall in provision is arguably the best way to bring about change and improvement with regard to the overall management of language-disordered children. A profile which demonstrates the child's progress on a graph, as discussed in Chapter 3, can be a useful visual way of making this clear to the rest of the team.

Treatment Ideas

An outline of the areas of difficulty experienced by language-disordered children in school has been provided within the assessment framework discussed in Chapter 2. This section deals with practical suggestions for primary and junior school children which can be implemented in the classroom. The speech therapists may wish to offer additional individual sessions or intensive group work during school holidays to work on particular aspects of language. When planning the timing of therapy for a particular child, the constraints of family life and the needs of the individual must be remembered. After-school appointments on dark, cold winter evenings may not be attended for a variety of reasons. Where clinic attendance is just not practical, the therapist may be better advised to concentrate efforts in the classroom. However, her or his ability to do so may be limited by district policy or an already full timetable. Before beginning classroom work with a language-disordered child, it is important to consider the underlying requirements for the child to progress in this environment.

Preparation for classroom learning: What is required?

Nearly everyone has a different view on what constitutes readiness to start school. Some parents may feel that the child should already be able to read and write his or her own name whilst the teacher may wish he or she could just do up a coat or put on shoes. When considering language and learning skills, it does seem that a great deal is expected of the average school entrant. For example, the child is required to assimilate verbal instructions whilst continuing with the task in hand. This assumes a fairly mature level of attention — at least level 5. If the group is large, the child may be further required to concentrate for longer periods and sustain or adapt an activity from instructions given to the group (this would be an attention level of 6), often in situations which include quite a high level of background noise. The grammatical complexity and length of the instructions will vary, making the example given at the beginning of this chapter more or less typical depending on the teacher's experience with language-disordered children. Various concepts and vocabulary will be encountered in the classroom which may not have been experienced at home or in the clinic, for example, the language of number work. Because most of the children will learn this new vocabulary quite quickly, it may be presumed that once it has been introduced it will not be necessary to repeat it subsequently.

Most language-disordered children can be expected to need more time to learn such material and recall it. It may also be assumed that the child will use previous knowledge, together with what is being learned in school, for problem solving. However, the language-disordered child will rarely manage to generalise his or her knowledge to the new situation. He or she will need opportunities to re-explore and confirm what he or she knows in the classroom situation.

Those children without language problems will be requesting information and commenting on their activities by this stage. This will allow them to report back on what they have been doing or ask for clarification if something is not understood. Language-disordered children will not usually have this range of pragmatic skills, except perhaps at a non-verbal level (using gesture, eye gaze or other body language to request attention or denote non-comprehension). Fluent and intelligible speech will also be the expected method of communication from children of this age. The average school entrant will possess most of these skills (Sheridan, 1977; Reynell, 1980). Moreover, teachers will be observing and monitoring progress in these areas during the first year of school. The language-disordered child will almost certainly fail to meet most, if not all, of these demands. However, it is possible, by working together, for teacher and therapist to facilitate situations in which these difficulties can be improved. Some of the basic requirements are discussed in the following section.

Attention and Listening Work

The integration of information the child receives by sight, sound and touch (even taste and smell!) are the fundamentals upon which learning is built. For the language-disordered child with auditory processing problems, work should begin with attention and listening. It is almost impossible to prepare the child for the distractibility and noise encountered in the school environment. However, it should be possible to build up his or her resistance to these factors before entry by using some of these techniques:

1. In the preschool speech therapy group, ask the child to complete a task while directing the others in something else.
2. Ask the child's family to send him or her on errands round the house or perhaps in the supermarket. Gradually aim to build up the child's tolerance and ability to deal with the interference of the television or radio and other family activities and conversations.
3. Ask the staff at the play group or nursery to give the child tasks to complete while other children are doing something else. Prepare a programme of activities which can be used beginning with simple non-verbal tasks, like matching or sorting, and progressing to carrying out commands and reporting back (about what he or she has done).

For the teacher, dealing with the very distractible child in the classroom can be time consuming and frustrating. Although it may be clear that the child needs more individual direction it may not be possible to provide this due to other demands. When this happens the child may rapidly move from one activity to another without accomplishing anything. In some children this may have been identified as immature behaviour. Others, with a more covert attention problem, may be considered to be daydreaming. It is important to describe the language-disordered child's difficulties accurately and devise methods of working on them in manageable units. This may best be done by using a checklist format, because teachers dealing with 20–30 children will need a quick and accurate way of recording their observations. Such a checklist for attention problems may look like the one below (with some examples provided):

Checklist for attention problems

1. Describe the child's level of attention: e.g. he or she works well at his or her choice of activity but when adult guidance is offered the child walks away.
2. Describe the different stages the child must gain to develop mature attention skills: e.g. stage 2 attention: the child will attend to his or her own choice of activity and not accept adult guidance.
3. Ask the teacher to describe some of the tasks he or she requires the child to carry out (keep the timescale of this short in order to make the targets reasonably attainable): e.g.
    Task one: draw round a template of a house.
    Task two: colour in the house in one colour.
    Task three: repeat task one and colour in roof and body of house in
                 different colours.
    Or for a group activity:
    The class listen to a story and then are given activity sheets. On these there are pictures which accompany the story. They have to fill in the missing details, parts of the pictures or key words from the board. The story is about building a house, so when the children have finished there is a choice of handling and weighing different building materials or drawing as many items as possible in the house which are made of wood.

In the group task the language-disordered child may not complete the first part of the activity and thus fail to understand the relevance of the second set of instructions. The next stage would be:

4. Devise a hierarchy which breaks down the complex task and offers practical suggestions. For the story task mentioned above this might be:
    The task: Did the child understand the story?
                 Did the child understand the instructions given?

If not, then either the use of pictures, a simpler explanation or a demonstration may help. If time is available actually begin the activity with the child.

Attention: Can the child finish the task sustaining attention right the way through?

Does the child find the teacher's comments or advice helpful or distracting?

Does the child find the comments and advice of other children helpful or distracting?

If not, then try to let him or her have a quieter place to work. Remember to give encouragement at key stages during the activity. Point out the next part of the task. Call his or her name if attention is wandering or he or she has moved away from the task. Cover up part of the page so that only one part of the task needs to be attended to at a time. If the words on the board are too far away from him or her to sustain attention, then provide a separate list. It is important, and therefore we continue to emphasise, that the child must find the task rewarding and experience success.

Once the teacher has become familiar with this type of checklist than a simpler one for more general use will be adequate. Here is an example:

Task:	*Description*
Skills involved:	1. Verbal comprehension of complex instructions
	2. Vocabulary
	3. Scanning and searching material
	4. Reading and writing
Strategies for coping:	1. Demonstration
	2. Repetition of instructions
	3. Simplification of task
	4. Additional picture clues
Levels of attention:	1. Working towards the task
	2. During the task
Strategies to overcome attention problems:	1. Physical proximity to adult
	2. Verbal direction by adult
	3. General encouragement

This basic framework can be further developed into more lengthy language programmes, some examples of which appear at the end of this chapter.

Introducing Teachers to the Scope of Language Disorders

Busy teachers will not have time to wade through vast amounts of information on language disorders. It is therefore important to consider how the subject can be presented in a succinct and comprehensive manner that is not oversimplistic. Initially, it may be better to confine descriptions of language problems to a particular child or group of children within his or her direct experience: begin with details about the child which are relevant to language development and continue by outlining the child's particular language skills in terms of strengths and weaknesses. Then examples should be given of when these have been observed in the classroom situation and their effect. From this description, it is possible to discuss the types of activities which could be carried out in the classroom. The following two cases (15 and 16) are examples of such descriptions to discuss with teachers.

Case 15

Background information: this boy was referred for speech therapy at the age of 2;6 years by the clinical medical officer who was concerned about his general development, as well as specifically about his speech and language development. There was no family history of developmental difficulties: both parents were healthy and employed in non-skilled labour, and a younger sister was developing normally. The medical officer observed a slight tremor in the right hand in fine motor tasks. The child had had two grand mal convulsions at 2 years but these were controlled with carbamazepine and there had been no further attacks. He had been admitted to a special opportunities nursery at the age of 3 years, but his attendance at speech therapy had been very irregular. At 4;6 years he was reassessed by the medical officer, and motor and social development were within the normal range. However, he had made little or no progress with speech and language. It was clear that he had difficulty with verbal comprehension. He had 6 months of regular speech therapy before he began school during which time the following problems were identified and worked on:

1. Comprehension and use of Wh questions.
2. Word-finding problem that required accessing relevant vocabulary both in comprehension and expression, and basic concepts for family and home life.

Strengths and weaknesses at school entry:

Strengths	Weaknesses
Attention:	
Generally good and accepts verbal direction	Loses it when he has problems with comprehension or word finding
Social:	
Considerate to peers, uses social phrases appropriately	Rather sensitive to failure

Strengths	*Weaknesses*
Comprehension:	
Relies on visual cues to understand the situation, will follow other's lead, copies peers when he doesn't understand, responds well to visual demonstration	He cannot respond to more abstract requests, e.g. 'What's this about?'
Sorting and classifying:	
When language is not used he can sort and classify items into groups but verbal instructions can confuse him. Visual demonstrations will help	Internal vocabulary is limited and he has problems with word retrieval to name groups and sets
Naming:	
He may get his meaning across by gesture	Will often use the wrong word for an item, even if it is quite well known
Response to questions:	
Will respond to some inverted questions, e.g. 'Are you 5?' Responds to forced alternatives like 'Can you eat it or wear it?' Also responds to mime, gesture and facial expression	Has specific non-comprehension of: Wh questions such as what, where, why and who, negatives such as 'the one not eating'; pronouns are muddled and so are tenses

This demonstrates the way in which general observation of behaviour can be mixed with more detailed descriptions of language problems as well as ideas for encouraging the child's development, and this gives the teacher a view of the problem which includes direct classroom observations. It covers a wide range of skills so that the teacher can see how this difficulty will fit into the various areas of the curriculum. A further example follows in Case 16.

Case 16

Background information: he was referred for speech therapy at 2;10 years of age by his health visitor. Birth, early development and feeding had not given cause for concern. He had had many episodes of asthma since the age of 9 months, and dribbling was constant during the initial assessment. He had very poor attention. He was an only child of an Arabic-speaking father and English-speaking mother, but only English was spoken in the home. Father was often absent from the family home, working overseas. The child joined a preschool language group at the age of 3 years, and listening and attention work was begun. At this stage, his verbal comprehension was formally assessed and found to be within the normal range. Three months later he joined a higher level group to begin work on expressive skills and more abstract concepts. At 3;6

years he was placed on review because expressive language was developing well. His mother requested further help with behavioural problems as he was often aggressive and destructive at home; he was seen by a clinical psychologist. The dribbling problem continued; he made considerable progress with expressive language, and by 4 years he was using question words and possessives. His attention was still rather unstable. His school entry was delayed by one term so that he could begin at 4;8 years. He received a period of intensive therapy aimed at increasing poor attention and listening and limited vocabulary; he was still dribbling. He had considerable difficulty with some concepts and basic sequencing skills, and had little idea of danger. He was often tearful when faced with direct language work, and his aggressive behaviour returned at home. Although he was recommended for language unit placement he had to wait several terms for this and continued to be seen in school during that time.

Strengths and weaknesses at 5 years:

Strengths	Weaknesses
Social:	
Engaging in good one-to-one relationships with well-known adults	Appears immature when compared with peers, often plays alone and is distractible. Can be aggressive
Comprehension:	
Is aware that he does not understand things but has no positive coping strategies It is easy to see when he is in difficulty; he whines, asks questions, refuses or cries	Comprehension is limited and vocabulary is patchy He has islands of ability but these are often not usable as he cannot organise or sequence information
Expression:	
This sounds good. Grammar is immature but within normal limits	There is little real information in what he says. Often struggles for specific words and may speak at a tangent to the subject. He has difficulties with more advanced grammar, muddling tenses and pronouns. Use of language is limited and he relies on adults to maintain the conversation

These two descriptions offer a good starting point for conversations with the teacher about the language-disordered child. Giving practical ways of working with these in the classroom is the next step; some of these ideas will be more appropriate for certain types of classroom learning than others.

Verbal Comprehension

When a large amount of information is given about a child, it may be difficult to prioritise this. It may be difficult to arrange much individual or small group work. As verbal comprehension is a vital constituent of learning in the classroom, it is usually a fundamental priority. When beginning to plan work for improving verbal comprehension with a teacher, it can be useful to introduce the concept of information-carrying words as described in Chapters 2 and 4 (Knowles and Masidlover, 1982). Other key strategies to discuss would be the use of gesture and/or additional visual cues. Monitoring the length and complexity of classroom instructions may be an initial difficulty for everyone. One way of considering this is to emphasise the effect of overcomplex instructions for that particular child. It may be that one child will panic and become very distracted, whilst another will just look bored and disinterested. Sharing these observations with the teacher allows modification of the instructions, depending on the reaction from the child. Here is an example of a typical request and some ways of modifying it:

> *Request*: Everyone, I want you to finish what you are doing now, but before you sit down, make sure your tables are tidy please.

Considerations:
1. Complexity of the instructions: in order to understand the complexity of this particular instruction, the child has to be able to understand an embedded clause: a before X do Y instruction. If the language-disordered child has not worked on before/after and first/next concepts, this will be confusing.
2. Use of vocabulary: it may not be clear who 'everyone' refers to. The child may not realise that this term actually includes him or her. He or she may only respond to directions given directly to him or her. Similarly 'finish' may not mean 'stop what you are doing' and 'tidy' may not mean 'put things away'.
3. Memory load: this instruction is long and includes very little redundant language which the child can ignore and still understand the sentence.
4. Pragmatic knowledge: the opening of the sentence 'everyone' goes on to presuppose that all the children will recognise that an important message follows. Shared knowledge of where to sit for the story is also presumed.

Having considered all of these points it would be possible to break down the sentence into smaller phrases and rearrange the essential elements of the message. It might become, 'Everyone finish now, tidy tables and sit down for story', which is only nine main elements. Or, if it is necessary to be more specific: 'Listen everyone, tidy your tables now. This table [point to table where child is working] put your pens in the box [wait for this to happen or repeat if necessary]. Listen children, are your tables tidy? [wait for response, verbal or non-verbal] Good, now sit here for a story [point].' In most cases it is possible to divide instructions into sections containing three or four information-carrying words or essential elements. Using key words such as 'listen' helps to alert the child to the instructions. Gestural cues help to reduce the verbal load even further.

Concepts and Vocabulary

An essential part of education is that children learn about things in a context and go on to apply this in various situations. Some of these situations will be known and others will be new. They will need to use this information to solve problems and make links between new areas of understanding. For example, the class is exploring the subject of clothes for the term. They are looking at the texture of materials, different uniforms worn in different occupations and the appropriate clothes for different environments. Most of the children in an infant class will be familiar with the vocabulary and concepts involved. The language-disordered child may be having considerable difficulty with the more abstract concepts, like 'silky' meaning 'smooth' or 'woolly' meaning 'warm'. He or she then has to make further links between these concepts and particular parts of clothing or uniforms. If this linking is done predominantly in words, the language-disordered child will be at a disadvantage. It will be easier for him or her if the actual clothing is available to help make these links. Actually helping the child to make links depends heavily on what the child already knows. It is important to build up from the well-understood and readily recognised concepts which are based on personal experience. Thus, with the subject of clothes, it is necessary to begin with the clothes the child wears in particular circumstances and the clothes family members or others in the immediate environment wear for different jobs. Once again the child's learning is based on success.

Organisational Problems

These problems are not always associated with language difficulty. They may be difficult to diagnose and require the combined experience of the teacher, educational psychologist, occupational and speech therapists. It is clear that some language-disordered children will have difficulties organising information (Gordon and McKinlay, 1980; Thomson, 1984). This may include difficulty in classifying information (e.g. situations and events) and making links between categories, particularly with concepts of time and space. It can also include difficulty with sequencing information, even recognising quite predictable sequences (like days of the week, or counting) and go on to include sequencing a series of events. Such children may also encounter difficulties in summarising information. For example, when a given outcome is stated, the child may have difficulty inferring what steps were taken to reach that end. Some children with organisational problems also have difficulties with physical coordination and actions, particularly undressing and dressing or manipulating craft materials. This may also interfere with the child's ability to find his or her way around the school. Case 17 is an example of a child with these types of difficulties.

Case 17

This boy was referred to speech therapy by his primary teacher. She was concerned about the increasing evidence of difficulty with language and learning as the child moved up through the infant and junior departments. He had been seen previously at the age of 3 years for speech therapy for a delay in speech and language developments. This appeared to have resolved quickly and was not apparent when he started school. By the end of his second year, he had made very little progress with reading. Despite a good visual memory, he had no strategy for encountering new written words, no knowledge of the phonic make up of words and very poor auditory sequencing skills. His drawing skills were excellent. His general level of vocabulary appeared satisfactory, but when put into situations which required specific recall, like 'what were we saying about tigers yesterday?', there was considerable evidence of word-finding difficulties. Expressive language contained some grammatical errors including difficulty with tenses and plurals. He was unable to recall the days of the week or the numbers 1–20 without repeating some in the sequence. He had difficulty using apparatus in science and maths sessions, so that it would all become jumbled and he would forget which piece served which function. In maths exercises, he would always need to use visual props like counting blocks. When aware of failure or pressure, he would often guess at an answer. He appeared anxious and was often tearful despite attempts to praise him and increase his self-confidence. After observing him and discussing his difficulties with his parents and teachers, a language programme was devised to involve work in clinic, home and school.

Children like this may be difficult to manage in the classroom situation, depending on how wide their organisational problems are. It is often difficult to decide on management priorities for a child with complex needs. Some of the key areas in which further work should lead to benefits for learning as a whole are outlined here.

Concepts of time and space

The child needs to know what day it is, what happens on particular days, how to find his or her way around the school etc. One one of working on this is to help the child to recognise predictable sequences of activity: begin with a typical part of the school day. When the child arrives follow a set sequence of events with him or her for taking off coats, sitting down, answering to name, beginning the first activity etc. This can be expanded to include larger sections of the day and week. Typical rotations of classroom activity should be included, for example, milk time is followed by story time. Visual aids may help the child grasp this. The child could have a personal picture calendar or diary to refer to which details these sequences.

Organising equipment

If a task requires a number of pieces of equipment which may become muddled, these could be arranged on a tray. Pictures which match each piece can help the child to replace it between parts of the activity so that he or she does not become confused about the function of each one or panic because all the bits are just piled in a heap on the table and he or she does not know where to start.

Summarising information

If the child is unable to cope with a general directive, it may be necessary to suggest ways in which it can be made more specific to the individual child. This may mean changing a general instruction like 'Tidy up' to 'put your pen away [wait until this is done], now put your book away'. Where the child is expected to be self-directed, for example, when getting ready to go out to play or getting changed for physical education (PE), then a child like this may require some direction. Again a personal chart of what needs to be done can help the child through such a sequence of actions.

Physical actions

The child's ability to actually carry out a sequence of actions will be important in organised games, PE, musical activities and craft work. For the more seriously impaired child, the advice of an occupational therapist will be essential. He or she will be concerned with observing the balance, coordination and sequencing required for each part of the activity being considered. Once again, the child's success will be important to the expected progress. Breaking actions down into smaller steps is a common strategy used for teaching action sequences. The action may need to be practised in a number of situations before moving on to a more complex skill.

Dealing with Expressive Difficulties

It may be useful to introduce the model proposed by Bloom and Lahey (1978) when discussing a child's expressive difficulties. This model is based on the interaction of three aspects of the child's language system: form (corresponding to syntax and phonology), content (semantics) and use (pragmatics). These three aspects of language are seen to interact to create the child's communicative potential. The terms 'form', 'content' and 'use' may be more accessible to other professionals. Once again, a checklist approach to documenting observations is recommended. Here is an example of the categories which would be included. The actual format would need to include space for the child's responses.

Checklist of expressive language observations

1. Language form:
    (a) single words;
    (b) relating two words together: nouns, verbs and adjectives;
    (c) stringing words together: short phrases, statements, comments, requests;
    (d) telegrammatic speech: note how the child marks grammatical inflections, tenses, plurals, regular and irregular, possession, negatives etc;
    (e) fluent speech; complex sentences.
2. Language content:
    (a) evidence of word-finding problems;
    (b) extent of basic vocabulary the child uses;
    (c) vocabulary specific to classroom situation: size, number, colour, shape, weight, height, comparisons;
    (d) vocabulary specific to subjects presently being taught, e.g. materials and texture for 'clothes' theme;
    (e) vocabulary for physical activities: direction and position;
    (f) vocabulary for social and emotional needs: sad, happy, angry etc.;
    (h) vocabulary for time and sequencing: days of the week, time of day, today, yesterday and tomorrow etc;
3. Language use:
    (a) range: statement, comment, request, teasing, humour, exclamation with both adults and children;
    (b) communication skills: methods used for gaining attention, initiating communication, knowledge of turn-taking, responding, maintaining a conversation.

(c) knowledge of self and others as communicators: the child's response to the rules of communication within specific contexts, with teachers, peers etc.

With a checklist system like this, the therapist and teacher can record observations quickly which can then be used as a basis for planning intervention strategies. The way in which a language programme can be developed for classroom use is best demonstrated by examples. Here are some sections of the language programmes developed for use with Cases 15 and 16, as referred to earlier. Both children were in the same class. The theme for the class for the term presented here was 'clothes'.

Classroom Language Programmes

Problems to work on

Specific comprehension problems

Case 15
This child cannot hold more than three information-carrying words in memory and process them for successful comprehension. Instructions need to be limited to account for this, e.g. 'Put the <u>pens</u> <u>in</u> the <u>box</u>'. He does not understand Wh questions which begin with why, who and where. He is unclear about negatives, e.g. 'the one not wearing socks'. He is unsure of possession, e.g. 'Teddy's coat', 'Get Jamie's shoe'.

Case 16
This child has listening and attention problems and poor comprehension. However, he could work at a level of three to four information-carrying words with Case 15 providing there was a minimum of distraction and adult help available, e.g. 'Find the <u>fireman's</u> <u>hat</u> and <u>gloves</u>'.

Ideas for working on these problems

1. Try to monitor the number of information-carrying words you use. If either child looks puzzled, you have probably used too many. Rephrase the sentence if possible. Split it into several shorter phrases. Add a gestural cue if all else fails.
2. Negatives and question forms: the children might dress up for different jobs or seasons. Provide photos to refer to so they can check what is correct for their given situation. For example, winter and summer clothes might allow for questions like: 'Is X cold? Is X hot? Who is cold? Who is hot?' Case 16 will need more gestural cues than Case 15.

A similar set of examples were constructed for word-finding problems as shown below.

Problems to work on

Word-finding problems

These are an expresssive difficulty due to an underlying problem in comprehending, storing and retrieving information.

Case 15 has a poor and unstable store of vocabulary. He only associates words with the function of objects at a very basic level. He often has difficulty retrieving them to use appropriately in sentences.

Case 16 has some small groups of vocabulary items which he knows well. However, these groups are often not related or used in different situations. He finds it difficult to make links between items and new situations.

Ideas for working on these problems

Help the children to cross-reference the different concepts so that clothes and season, clothes and people, clothes and jobs, clothes and family members, clothes and time of day, become better connected for them. Use real clothes where possible and set them out in correct sets. Gradually mix them up so that one item in the set is wrong. Work from concepts they already know like clothes for boys vs girls, hot vs cold before introducing new ones like thick and thin. Try to use the real clothes to act out situations from the children's recent experiences, e.g. going on holiday. Begin with clothes they did need and go on to introduce ones that are not relevant. An 'odd one out game' can be developed first using clothes, and then in picture form. Ask the children to show and explain, both verbally and non-verbally, which is the odd one out of the set.

In this way, a language programme could go on to include other relevant areas of strengths and weaknesses depending on the amount of attention the teacher can devote to the individual children. Do not try to suggest too many things at once. It is better to concentrate on a few areas and achieve the goals set than suggest too many so that none are done in any detail. The other aspects of work mentioned in this chapter – concept development, attention and listening, expressive language etc. – could be added in a similar way. Keep a consistent structure to the programme so that it can be followed easily. Remember to give specific examples of the activities suggested. 'Dressing up' is a well-known activity and will require no further explanation. Where activities are not generally known, then take time to demonstrate what you mean. It is better to try to use activities common to the classroom than to introduce too many new ones. What is unfamiliar practice is unlikely to be adopted in a busy situation. Take time to monitor response to the programme. If possible, use another checklist on which observations about the child's response to activities can be recorded. Make sure that you return, evaluate the effectiveness of the programme and plan the next step.

As the child moves from primary to junior school age, so the opportunites to use visual cues and direct experience diminish. It becomes increasingly important for the child to work from written instructions either from the board, a book or worksheets (Pocklington and Hegarty, 1982). As the child tries to cope with increasingly heavy language demands, the size of the class, the opportunity for individual work with the teacher and the level of background noise may all play a part in the child's success or failure at a task. However, there are some strategies which can be adopted to help children who are having difficulty in a mainstream junior or middle school in these circumstances. For the child to continue to succeed he or she must be able to do the following.

Understand classroom instructions

As the grammar and vocabulary become more complex the child must develop the skill of attending to the key words and disregarding what is redundant information. The previous discussion about simplifying classroom instructions may be just as relevant here. The child must also be encouraged to seek help if necessary or ask for a repetition of instructions.

Learn from a text and understand written instructions

Whilst the language-disordered child's concept of number may be better developed, he or she may fail at mathematics tasks due to the written language of worksheets or text books. The written instructions may be complex or confusing. Here the child needs to learn to identify the key words in the text. Initially, it may help to underline these to draw the child's attention to them. Then he or she can be encouraged to develop this strategy for him- or herself.

Infer and share knowledge from one situation to another

More and more, inference and sharing of knowledge about the environment, the world, individuals etc. are assumed rather than stated. For example this sentence: 'Let's look at the face and hands, remember we're doing quarters, past and to: where do the hands go?' can be very confusing until you realise the subject is 'telling the time'. Seemingly abrupt changes of topic and reference take place. Previous information is referred back to and the language-disordered child may miss much of this.

One way of working on these kinds of problem is to divide the lesson plan into essential (core) knowledge and non-essential (additional) information. In this way it is easier to monitor what the language-disordered child must learn, what he or she has learned, so that it can be built on and generalised, and what is optional or extra.

When language-disordered children enter school they often seem to disappear, not necessarily due to the overwhelming success of language remediation programmes, but as a result of the lack of follow-up studies monitoring the progress of language-disordered children in mainstream school (Urwin, Cook and Kelly, 1988). More work is needed to describe accurately the classroom conditions in terms of the language that is used and the way this is used. The ideas mentioned here aim to provide a basis for the cooperative working of teachers and therapists. Successful joint working of this kind will require considerable commitment by both parties as well as the on-going support of service managers. Not all language-disordered children will be reabsorbed into the peer group without further reference to their language problems at a later stage. There will be those who continue to experience different difficulties with language in their teens, and it is the needs of this group which are discussed in the next chapter.

Chapter 6
Teenagers with
Language Disorders

Summary

The educational and social needs of language-impaired teenagers are discussed. Clinical examples are discussed together with the results of some research studies. There is an emphasis on the use of group work which should aim towards social competence and independence.

Introduction

Very little has been written specifically about teenagers with language disorders, their problems and needs. In the early stages of diagnosis and assessment most parents ask about the long-term implications of language difficulty, but there are few detailed studies from which to draw information. Ripley and Lea (1984) have provided one of the few studies to have followed up a group of severely language-disordered school leavers and to document their attainments. They presented information from case histories of 23 subjects who had attended a school for severely speech and language-disordered children (both developmental and acquired disorders). All the children had a diagnosis of severe receptive aphasia, and there were 13 males and 10 females: four were married (three males and one female) and three had children (two males and the female).

At the time of follow-up, 20 of the subjects were in full-time paid employment (one was re-training and the status of two was unknown). In terms of other social adjustments, it was difficult to make objective measures. Three of the group said they attended social clubs for the deaf and nine held a driver's licence. Most of them said they used speech to communicate, although two had virtually no speech and four had very limited speech. Signing and finger spelling were also used to communicate when necessary, usually to clarify what had been said rather than as a replacement for speech. The majority of those who were unmarried continued to live with their parents or under their supervision (although this could not be described as unusual among this age group); only time will tell if independence is achieved by these young people. Those who were married with young families were described as showing 'a remarkably modern attitude towards role sharing' (Ripley and Lea, 1984, p. 21).

Studies of less severely language-disordered teenagers in mainstream, rather than special, education are non-existent. However, most parents and clinicians will recognise that the transition to secondary education represents a particularly large hurdle for even a mild to moderately impaired child. The language demands of most secondary education, identified 20 years ago by Barnes (1969), are considerable. Yet few secondary schools have either the resources or the experience to accommodate language-impaired children adequately. Clearly, the pupil must be able to integrate a wide range of information and communication provided in a number of different modalities (spoken or written, by computers, in debates, through drama or poetry and in foreign languages, to name a few) and presented by a number of different teachers each with an individual style. This must then be processed and understood in order that it may be represented in an equally wide range of forms, including spoken and written examinations. No wonder that a number of language-impaired children, previously unidentified, surface at this stage.

Barnes (1969) emphasises the way in which teachers need to be aware of the language they use in the classroom. This advice applies equally to therapists and to others working with language-impaired children. We need a greater awareness of the way in which language-impaired teenagers are isolated within the curriculum and social life of the school, including the way in which the use of specialist terminology is particularly isolating. A successful life in secondary school is considerably influenced by the young person's ability to use questions to gain information, yet some may have considerable difficulty with this format. We need to explore other ways of making information available to them including encouragement to 'think out loud' as well as non-verbal expression. The language policy across the curriculum, which forms the conclusions of Barnes, Britton and Rossen (1969), concludes with a statement about the role of the teacher in the classroom which, from experience, seems to ring true for all those concerned about the communicative potential of teenagers. They emphasise the need for the teachers (and we would add all others) to be prepared to work alongside the pupils. This is more likely to develop initiative and confidence in the pupils' use of language as well as encouraging a more creative and less stereotyped form of language. For such a model to be implemented, much more multidisciplinary working will be required in our secondary schools. Teachers, speech therapists and parents need to work together to understand the language needs of language-disordered children. They need to recognise each others' skills and collaborate in producing programmes which meet the children's need for a language that is useful for life.

To date, research in speech and language development has paid little specific attention to the language of teenagers. Whilst it is clear that, in normal children, the major hurdles of the early years have been overcome by this stage, the refining of the language system to cope with the increasingly complex demands of adult usage goes on. The implications of this 'fine tuning' for the language-impaired teenager are rarely discussed, and these authors have met a marked reluctance among therapists to engage in language remediation tasks with teenagers. Most of this reluctance is probably related to the clinical dilemma already discussed (Coombes, 1987) of 'How to know what to do' etc. Some of the features of language development characteristic of the teenage years are discusssed by Wiig (1987). She emphasises the fact that, from the age of 9 to 16 years, the major change to the way in which language is used is in relation to problem solving. This is brought about first through an increasing knowledge of vocabulary and concepts, an awareness of their multiple meaning and use of the semantic relations which can be expressed by combining these. Secondly, the user, through social maturity, gains an improved sociolinguistic awareness and knowledge such that he or she can switch between linguistic codes and take account of the different perspectives of the speaker and listener. Thirdly, there is an increasing ability to relate spoken information to past experiences and internalised knowledge as well as to make inferences. Finally, there is a growing ability to analyse the words, phrases and sentences that are employed both by the individual and by others. This complex set of abilities would appear to interact and contribute to the potential linguistic competence of adulthood. The language-disordered teenager clearly faces a much harder task in trying to achieve this competence through the integration of this range of skills.

Problems with language may initially present as something else. A lot of mild but non-specific health problems which keep the child away from school frequently, a failure to complete homework, an increase in aggressive behaviour or a failure to integrate with peers may be a sign of an underlying language problem. Of course, this multiplicity of things may also be unrelated to language difficulty. Once again, the need for comprehensive assessment and differential diagnosis by a multidisciplinary team must be emphasised. Some of the language assessment techniques which are suitable for the age range 11−18 are discussed in Chapter 2. Whilst they are predominantly from the USA (which makes some test items rather culturally exclusive), their sensitive use does reveal useful diagnostic information. Some clinicians will prefer to use a battery of different tests to create a language profile, as discussed in Chapter 3. Once again, the difficulty here is that few tests specifically cover this age range.

However, some tests can be recommended from clinical experience. To produce a language profile similar to that discussed in Chapter 3 the following are recommended:

1. For auditory verbal comprehension: the Test for Reception of Grammar (Bishop, 1983).
2. For confrontational naming: the Graded Naming Test (McKenna and Warrington, 1983) for which preliminary norms for children aged 11–14 years are available (Lees, 1989).
3. For sentence repetition, and some other subtests: the Spreen–Benton Neurosensory Examination of Aphasia. Although this test was designed for adults, Gaddes and Crockett (1975) have produced norms for children aged 6–13 years.
4. For those who prefer a comprehensive test battery in one package the Clinical Evaluation of Language Functions (CELF; Semal and Wiig, 1987) is frequently recommended for this age group.

When a teenager is referred for assessment, the concerns of parent and child do need to be taken seriously. Where possible the young person should be invited to contribute equally to the discussion about areas of difficulty, particular strengths, strategies already used and motivation for further intervention. The benefits of a multidisciplinary team cannot be sufficiently emphasised. Whilst the direct contribution that the medical members of the team could make may have diminished, unless there are new or ongoing developments that suggest otherwise (epilepsy for example), the combined contribution of all the team members, particularly the educational psychologist, is important in producing a comprehensive view. From clinical experience the following questions are often asked about the language difficulties of teenagers.

Which School is Best for the Child Now?

Whilst the statementing procedure which is a provision of the 1981 Education Act is primarily for the benefit of individual children and is supposed to reflect their specific needs, it has become a minefield for many parents and professionals. Rather than concentrating on providing for the individual needs of children, all too often the procedure has been seen to reflect the political manoeuvring of education authorities and the personal insecurities of the various professionals involved. Many parents find the procedure lengthy, exhausting and complex, despite the information provided by education departments and organisations concerned for children with special needs. However, when the procedure works well, some creative and productive ways of providing for the educational needs of language-impaired teenagers can result. It is difficult to know how many language-impaired teenagers would benefit from a statement of educational needs. In Lees' (1989) study of children with acquired aphasia (which is further discussed in Chapter 9), 14 of the 34 children were teenagers. At the time of writing, six of these have statements of educational need; three of these are in special education placements and three are in mainstream school.

It is not uncommon for a child to be referred for a second opinion or further assessment at the time of transition from primary to secondary school. This often reflects the anxieties of family and teachers about the child's ability to manage within mainstream education when it is so demanding. However, it is often unclear what alternatives would best suit the child's needs, and only comprehensive assessment will help to clarify this. Case 18 presented for assessment in this respect and demonstrates some of the complexities of cases of this kind.

Case 18

This child was 11;5 years old when she was referred for a speech therapy assessment by the paediatric neurologist to whom she had recently been referred by her GP. The parents' major concern was about her future schooling, but she clearly had a range of difficulties well known to her teachers. These included clumsiness in fine and gross motor skills, poor auditory and visual memory and sequencing skills, as well as difficulties in verbal comprehension, word finding and use of complex sentences. She was left-handed and had been adopted in the first month of life. She was described as a rather socially isolated and timid child.

Speech and language assessment on two occasions suggested a fluctuating receptive language disorder, which was consistent with reports of her ability at home and school. She had difficulty with the speed of auditory verbal processing and needed a number of repetitions of test instruction on the TROG. There was evidence of difficulty of recall of words in confrontational naming and association naming tasks as well as in conversation. She did not appear over-anxious in the test situation and was able to discuss her difficulties at a simple level. She said she was unhappy that she had no friends at school and no one to visit after school hours. Pure-tone audiometry confirmed normal hearing. The paediatric neurologist reported a normal physical examination. An EEG showed an occasional burst of abnormal activity in the right hemisphere, predominantly in the temporal and parietal lobes. She had no history of seizures.

It was clear from a school visit that the high level of language processing required even in the primary school classroom was beyond her capacity most of the time. Whilst it might have been possible, if individual help were available, for her to have remained there, it was clear that the level of receptive language ability required in mainstream secondary school would be unlikely to be met by such provision. She was therefore placed in a small mixed tutorial unit where individual and small group work was possible, and where speech therapy and occupational therapy could also be added to the curriculum.

This is just one example of the way in which receptive language disorders and auditory verbal processing problems can interrupt classroom learning. Not all children with this type of difficulty would require special provision. Case 21 from Chapter 9 (a girl with an acquired aphasia) had a residual high level problem of this nature. She remained in mainstrean school with a personal tutor who would help with comprehension tasks, both within the classroom and in individual sessions. Thus she was able to go through verbal instructions with the tutor when they were first given and go through them again before working through her own homework. This tutor was also available to work in cooperation with the speech therapist on building up the child's self-monitoring and self-cueing skills. Three years after the onset of her aphasia, she no longer needed an individual tutor in the classroom, although she continued to have access to one for individual sessions as required. She had developed the capacity to cue herself in tasks involving complex instructions by breaking down the senetence and repeating it in pieces to check her own comprehension. Although this made her work slower than her peers, she was sufficiently accurate. She gained considerable confidence from working with her tutor and was well integrated with her peers. She passed three GCSEs at the age of 16 years. This is an example of the way in which difficulties of this kind can be managed within mainstream education when resources are available and professionals work together.

Will the Child be able to do Public Examinations?

The development of the GCSE examinations has theoretically made it easier for language-disordered teenagers to gain such qualifications before leaving school. These examinations can be taken at many different levels and include provision for continuous assessment for the pupil's work throughout the course. In this way not all of the emphasis is placed on the pupil's performance on the day of the examination. This is an important consideration for language-disordered teenagers, even those with quite high level problems, whose language skills often suffer under the pressure of time. Comprehension may require some further repetition, and word finding will involve a greater degree of search and hesitation. Neither of these problems means that language-disordered teenagers cannot do examinations; rather they emphasise the need for the school to have a clear idea of how the language disorder will affect the pupil's ability to cope under examination conditions. Extra time within the examination to allow for the effects of difficulties in speed and volume of verbal processing and recall can then be arranged. It is also possible to arrange for someone to read the question paper to the pupil where written comprehension is slower, or in some way more impaired, than auditory comprehension.

The subjects which a language-disordered teenager takes for examination need careful consideration and discussion along with all aspects of vocational guidance. It will be important to counsel the pupil sensitively about career choice. However, having a language disorder does not preclude the child taking, for example, English or other subjects with a heavy language load, particularly where continuous assessment is part of the course. Studying a second language may be more problematic. Careful account should be taken of the demands made on these pupils by an oral examination, which will probably require extra preparation time at the very least. It is also important that the pupil in a mainstream school should not feel singled out by these measures to create equality of opportunity within the examination system. Open discussion with the individual about this is essential. Moreover, there are quite likely to be a number of other pupils who also have special needs which require consideration (eyesight problems, learning difficulties of various kinds).

It is difficult to establish how many language-disordered teenagers go on to take public examinations. Of the 14 already mentioned in the Lees (1989) study of acquired aphasia (see Chapter 9), 4 had already passed between 3 and 10 subjects at GCE or GCSE level and a further 4 were studying for others. It is important that we document long-term follow-up of language-impaired children so that a clearer view of their possible educational attainments can be obtained. This will be valuable when discussing further educational opportunites with pupils and families.

Will the Child be able to live as an Independent Adult?

Independent living is a particular concern for all parents of children with special needs. It is usually a consideration which needs planning for earlier rather than later. Where the family works towards independent living as a goal right from the start, it is more readily achieved than where the issue is avoided until the late teens. There is no fundamental reason to suggest that even a severely language-disordered young adult cannot live independently, as can be seen from the Ripley and Lea (1984) study.

However, it is clear that some specific considerations may be required. First, the language-disordered teenager may be slower to mature socially than non-language-impaired peers. This may lead to their being treated as a younger child and to expectations being lowered in respect of their possible adult achievements. It may mean that they have difficulty forming close relationships, particularly with a view to marriage or other long-term relationships. They may look for an older person as a mentor, advisor or counsellor. It may be important to search out appropriate social groups where they can feel comfortable and valued group members. Vocational guidance will need to be sensitive and informed. It may be helpful for such young people to attend further education or training courses, both to obtain vocationally relevant qualifications and to act as a transition from school to work.

Once again it is difficult to know how many severely language-disordered children get jobs and what types of occupations these are. In the fourteen teenagers previously mentioned in Lees (1989), three have left school at the time of writing: one employed as a greengrocer's assistant and two on youth training schemes (one for hairdressing and one for catering). Three of the others opted to continue their education after the age of 16 years in order to study for further examinations.

Where signing is still a major part of the communication system of a language-impaired teenager it is important to consider the social and employment implications of this. Ripley and Lea (1984) recommend that all their severely language-disordered young people should register as disabled when leaving school, although not all do this. Support from the disablement resettlement officer in the area where the young person lives and works can be valuable in helping to make the adjustments from school to work and independent living. Social activities, particularly clubs for the deaf, have also been mentioned as a possible place of contact for young people with language disorders, particularly those still heavily reliant on signing.

The Association for all Speech Impaired Children (AFASIC) is concerned with helping young people adjust to independent living. From a very young age, members of AFASIC can take part in appropriate activities which are designed to build self-esteem, foster independence and motivation, and social integration. These include outdoor activites, such as canoeing and mountaineering, as well as hobbies like photography. A newsletter keeps members in touch with each other, and they are able to meet up at a number of venues and activities throughout the year. Recently, AFASIC has also tried to encourage young people with language disorders to try a broader range of activities. In this respect a small group of young people and adults have been on a journey to the USA. It should be remembered that the voluntary sector makes an important contribution to the life in the community for young people with language disorders.

Equipping the Language-impaired Child with a Language for Life

In her discussion of the transitions in language skill which takes place in the teenage years, Wiig (1987) emphasised the importance of metalinguistic abilities. She stated that whilst most of these metalinguistic skills develop during middle childhood, some appear in the period 8–13 years of age. They include an ability to intepret ambiguous sentences, figurative language, jokes and sarcasm, and using language to plan written and oral production as, for example, in decision making. Language-impaired young people who fail to develop these skills tend to use a range of other strategies to overcome this gap in their language development. They may use the most common interpretation or inference, or base a response solely on personal experience (Wiig and Secord, 1986). When interpreting metaphorical expressions this tends to be done literally. In conversational situations, timing of responses is often poor so that he or she will either respond too quickly without taking sufficient time to reflect, or respond after a significant delay indicating difficulty in processing and/or recall.

This range of difficulties can be a significant problem in many important situations the young person will meet on leaving school, such as a job interview or trying to take a driving test. Earlier discussion of the use of metalinguistic skills in helping the young language-disordered child to grasp concepts associated with the phonological system (see page 117), does suggest that it is possible to make language more tangible to young people with language difficulties. It is important to give relevant and clear feedback about communicative efficiency, first in a controlled environment and later in a range of natural situations. Three techniques can be useful in this respect. The first is the value of group work. A small group of three or four young people who have already established a good peer relationship can provide a helpful environment in which to explore aspects of interpersonal communication. It is important to balance the group and know the strengths and weaknesses of all the members before beginning a programme. A group in which all the members are either too verbal and competitive or too reticent and passive is unlikely to be successful. Where one member has good non-verbal skills, another may have better comprehension or vocabulary, and these skills can be shared in a group situation. The adult must be prepared to be a full member of the group. In this respect, it is not always necessary for the adult to be the group leader. As the competence of the group members increases, it is useful to allow others to experience this role for themselves.

The use of role-playing within the group is the second thing to consider. The group may begin by discussing situations suggested by the adult and then trying to re-enact these. Later, as the competence of the group develops, real situations encountered by the individuals concerned can be discussed and re-enacted. Picture material can be ambiguous and poorly interpreted by young people with pragmatic difficulties. It is necessary to make sure that what is used is clear; photographs may be preferable. The realism and relevance of the situation is also important. Whilst it might seem fun to discuss how to explain directions to a character from a science fiction film, it is probably more useful to consider first of all the problem in respect of the kind of person who might be met in the street.

When working on role-playing, the therapist should ensure that the actual incident does not go on for too long. Poor memory skills may limit the amount the young people can realistically retain and later discuss. Where necessary, particularly in the initial stages, props to help memory and sequence of action can be useful. If the group has reasonable written language skills, captions can also be used to aid recall. Whilst role-playing is a valuable technique, it does not suit everbody. Some young people may find it very difficult and rather pressurising. The group will need to be handled sensitively when anxieties become apparent. Anxiety may be based on lack of self-esteem or experience of failure, either in the present group or in a previous one. It is important to continue to base therapy, even at this stage, on the individual teenager's experience of success. However, the therapist's enthusiasm for the situation should not overwhelm the group so that it is no longer helpful to them.

So much can be happening in a group working on pragmatic skills, that it is difficult to keep track of it all; feedback is very important in these activities. We also need to bear in mind the need for continual re-evaluation of the progress of the group and the individuals in it. Therefore a video camera and recorder can be a vital piece of equipment. The opportunity to rewind the action or pause at a particular moment can be useful for picking up on an example of a specific skill or sequence of skills. It is also good to use the video to point out examples of successful communication when these are achieved.

However, it is possible that a young person with a language disorder will have significant, or at least some, difficulty in communication on leaving school. This may have a continued effect on self-esteem and social integration. Such a difficulty may motivate the young person to seek further therapy as an adult. The most important thing to consider when meeting such an individual is the need for open and realistic discussion about the possible improvements that any further therapy might lead to.

Human communication is actually infinitely variable in the adult; each person has a unique system which is flexible and creative and through which he or she can interact with others. This enormous variety means that people's use of language varies, and even varies for each individual depending on the situation. Some people are just more verbal. Whilst we should aim to develop the full potential of the language-disordered individual, we also need to remember that complex verbal language is not the norm for everyone. A therapy programme which has emphasised success at each stage of development should lead to a well-adjusted individual who is able to make the best of both strengths and weaknesses in adult life.

Chapter 7
Where to go from here

Summary

Methods of collecting, organising and presenting data are outlined with a view to developing research techniques. Clinical caseloads and management strategies are described. A flexible approach is adopted which attempts to maximise staff expertise and resources, while keeping the children's needs a central issue.

There is clearly a great deal of work which goes beyond the direct treatment and management of the children and which contributes to our further understanding of language disorder. Unless we are prepared to explore where our clinical practice, critical evaluation and discussion are leading, we will not develop new models and ideas about language development and disorder. Some will feel that models and ideas are for other people and are not the domain of the clinician. We would disagree, as our experience confirms that such exploration sharpens clinical practice. In this chapter, we shall consider a range of ways of working with language-disordered children and/or collecting and presenting information about them.

Speech therapists often work alone and may seldom have the opportunity to meet and discuss particular cases and treatment strategies beyond the local level. They probably spend hours recording information in case notes and devising language programmes and equipment that are never shared with others (Crystal, 1982b). Being clinically effective is also about how to collect information and share it with other people. A reluctance to engage in such tasks is often attributed to lack of time, lack of experience in any particular field and problems in deciding how to organise and record information. A failure to assume responsibility for this aspect of professional development relegates much of the valuable work that is produced in clinics to heaps of files which continually gather dust. For example, where a clinician has amassed a wealth of detail about a language-disordered child, it remains in the form of an opinion rather than being transferred to a written description which could then be used for discussion and comparison. The methods presented here for dealing with clinical data have been developed and recommended from personal experience.

Some Methods of Collecting Data

Obviously, good working practice demands that a clear written account is kept of all aspects of the speech therapy contact with any child. Therefore,

Name: Diagnosis	TROG A	RDLS	WFVT	GNT	Aud. assoc.	Sent. rep.	Story	Reading
Date of birth: Handedness:								
Assessment 1 Date: CA								
Comments:								
Assessment 2 Date: CA								
Comments:								
Assessment 3 Date: CA								
Comments:								
Assessment 4 Date: CA								
Comments:								

Figure 7.1   Sample data sheet for results for language-disordered children

all clinicians record facts like test scores and descriptions of observation. However, this is often done in a haphazard way so that returning to the case notes at a later date, or worse still when a colleague tries to do so, it is difficult or sometimes impossible to find or understand the information required. Some ways of making these notes more effective are given below.

The use of formal assessments

Most therapists will use formal tests at some time during the child's development. These will allow him or her to monitor the child's progress over time and in comparison with peers. This is usually done by making an age-equivalent comparison with chronological age. We have already outlined how to use the z-score calculation (p. 82) in order to compare scores across tests and consider rates of progress over time. Even so understanding the child's progress can be further enhanced by displaying this information so that it can be interpreted at a glance. A summary sheet which records all test scores can be kept at the front of the notes. An example of this kind of sheet is given in Figure 7.1. A copy of this sheet can be kept with those obtained for other children in order to facilitate cross-child comparisons between similar types of language disorders. The data can be transferred to graphs, which can then be shared with colleagues in discussions. An example of the type of graph used in this book, which has proved very useful in practice and research, is given in Figure 7.2. These can both be adapted to include whichever test information is preferred.

Clinical evaluation of progress

The clinician may wish to compare the broad trends in progress made by individuals or groups of children who take part in different treatment programmes. Whilst these are not intended to replace the more stringent methods discussed in Chapter 8, they can be used to evaluate the future direction of the present programme. To begin with the clinician must select the types of communication which will be recorded for this evaluation. This might simply be the absence or presence of a particular skill during a part of the treatment session, such as the use of two-word utterances. The next question is to decide on an appropriate way to record these observed behaviours. This may mean counting the numbers which occur in part of a session (which may need to be taped or video-taped unless an observer can do the recording live). From this point, it is possible to show that, at the beginning of the therapy period, the child used no two-word utterances in therapy session, but by a certain point in the programme he or she was producing them in every session.

·Such a system can then be augmented with other ways of quantifying the child's responses. A rating scale of 1–5 could be used to describe the

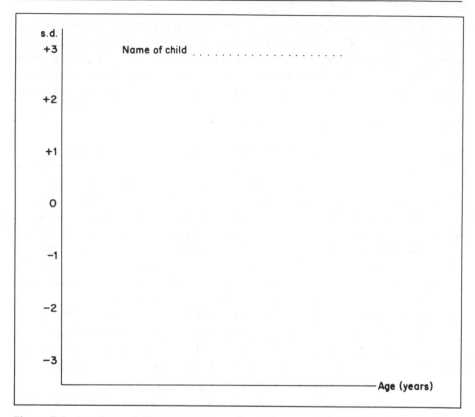

Figure 7.2 Sample graph. T = Test for Reception of Grammar; W = Word Finding Vocabulary Test; S = Sentence Repetition; A = Association Naming

child's responses so that the numbers stand for the frequency of occurrence of the behaviour:

> 0: the child never uses the behaviour
> 1: the child occasionally uses the behaviour
> 2: the child sometimes uses the behaviour
> 3: the child uses the behaviour about half of the time
> 4: the child uses the behaviour most of the time
> 5: the child uses the behaviour all the time

Because this is a subjective scale, it will be necesary to decide what the terms 'occasionally' and 'sometimes' mean in a specific context. This is particularly important if the scale is used with parents or other professionals. It can be quite useful to have such a scale for home or school visits as it makes recording observations much quicker. It is also important to remember that this is not an interval scale (i.e. the transition between numbers 2 and 3 it not necessarily equal to that between 4 and 5). The numbers merely serve to summarise a set of observations about the child.

Another way of approaching this problem is to take a base 10 approach (Fawcus et al., 1983). This entails devising a number of assessment activities which can be repeated at regular intervals during the treatment programme, but which are not the treatment tasks. Each activity is comprised of 10 test items which require a similar level of skill in order to score correctly, e.g. 10 picture cards of familiar actions which the child has to label with the correct verb or 10 commands which are of similar complexity. The tasks are presented at intervals during the treatment programme, e.g. the beginning of each week for 6 weeks. The child scores 1 to 10 on the assessment task depending on how many of them are correct. Sampling behaviour in this way allows effective monitoring of progress. The numerical information can be transferred directly to a summary graph for quick reference.

Observation checklists

It can be useful to use a checklist in a wide range of situations to allow for a comparison of the child's behaviour. There are a number available which are outlined in Chapter 2 (Bzoch and League, 1970; Gerard, 1986), but these may be rather long, depending on the situation. When working in a small group with other professionals, it can be helpful to have a checklist on which the child's behaviour during a session can be recorded. It will be necessary to give a brief description of each behaviour so that the task can be completed quickly. For example, a checklist to record the level at which the child's attention control was during a number of sessions might look like this:

Rating scale: 0 = never, 1 = sometimes, 2 = 50% of time 3 = always.

Attention:	Date	Date	Date	Date
	3.10	4.10	5.10	6.10
Level 1: highly distractible	3	2	2	1
Level 2: single channelled	0	1	1	2

and so on through other levels and dates as appropriate.

A simple rating scale will once again convert descriptive information to numerical scores. These can then be analysed later for trends and progress.

Video record

Communication is such a complex skill that often a video recording will be the best way to assess some areas, particularly pragmatic skills. A video record taken over time can be a useful way of showing progress to parents and other staff. If more objective information is required, then it will be necessary to view it with a colleague and see if a rating scale can reliably be agreed on. The use of video-taping in therapy sessions is becoming more available. Several basic points must be remembered if a recording is going to be used to document progress, including the fact that the subject must be clearly seen and heard. There is no point presenting a video in which the child's speech is more indistinct or unintelligible than in real life. This can take quite a bit of practice before good results are achieved.

Surveys

The people who are on the receiving end of the child's communication, i.e. the parents and teachers, can be asked for observations about the child's progress. Gathering opinions which are then useful for suggesting trends in progress in a group of children can be quite a complex procedure. Obvious pitfalls include ambiguous questions and many different forms of experimental bias according to the way the questions are set out and the answers recorded. Questions should not be phrased in such a way that the respondent knows the answer the questioner is seeking from the format of the question; this can happen if there is only one choice of response given. The respondent may also misunderstand what is required because the format is unclear. It is often difficult to see these errors when working alone and it may be worth while asking someone with more experience (most health/education authorities have a 'research department') to help in the planning of any survey.

As a general point, the collecting and organising of data should not be particularly time consuming or call for radical changes in practice or it will defeat its purpose. Once score sheets and checklists have been drawn up the clinician should soon develop the habit of recording the score(s). The next step is to consider how to use all the data that have been accumulated. Formal research designs are recorded in the next chapter. Less formal methods of using data include discussions at case conferences, study or support groups or formal presentations at lecture or conference level. The primary factor is to present the case coherently so that the members of the group/audience are clear about what has been said. Some ways of ensuring this are:

1. Additional visual information usually makes comprehension easier than auditory information alone. It may therefore be appropriate to produce a handout detailing the main points or specific examples.
2. When discussing treatment procedures, give a full and thorough description: who did what, where and for how long. Very little is written about the structure and activity of therapy sessions and this has led to a vague notion of what therapy really is. If we want to discuss whether or not it is effective, we have to know what actually took place.

3. Become familiar with any technical equipment, video player, slide or overhead projector, before you start the presentation/discussion.

4. If presenting slides or acetates with diagrams or words, remember to keep them simple. A visual aid which contains too much information is no aid at all.

5. Be aware of using exclusive jargon or terminology. If it is unavoidable make sure you explain it.

6. Give practical and real examples where possible.

7. Do speak clearly and confidently. Do not spend the whole talk apologising for what you did or thought. Describe the reasons for your decisions, but also state when you are being subjective or intuitive.

8. Where at all possible, go through the presentation/discussion with a colleague beforehand. This helps to ensure that it will be clear and increases self-confidence. It can help you to identify areas likely to require further discussion or about which questions will be asked.

9. Remember timing and do not overrun any time limits as the group/audience will lose interest.

10. Bear in mind that there will be questions and criticisms. This is not a reason for avoiding such presentations. The only way we will make progress professionally is by discussion and constructive criticism of models and ideas.

Keeping abreast of developments in the area of language disorder is not always easy for busy clinicians. Terminology seems to change and new research is constantly being reported in a host of journals. Ways of keeping up with current literature, and new assessment and treatment methods, will be important to those working with language-disordered children. When looking at a new paper about language disorder read the summary first and see if you want to look at it in detail or just skim through on the basis of what is briefly outlined. If you do decide to read more, get a broad idea of the method and then concentrate on the discussion of the results and what they mean. It is important to see the results in context. Language-disordered children present as a heterogeneous group and therefore the results from a small group with phonological problems cannot necessarily be extrapolated to a larger group with, for example, receptive difficulties. Discussing recent papers in a support group can help to clarify their relevance for your own clinical practice. For those already qualified, remember the value of a student therapist to the department. He or she will, hopefully, be learning up-to-date information and perhaps have access to new assessment material. Student placement is not all about what the clinician can teach the student, but more realistically about a reciprocal exchange of ideas that benefits both parties.

Occasionally there are specific areas that a clinician wishes to explore further, as the result of attending a course or when a group of similar children are referred. Many regions now have interest groups which meet formally (some under the auspices of the College of Speech Therapists) or informally to exchange information and ideas. With the increasing diversity of speech therapy and the pace of new developments in language disorder, membership of such groups is to be highly encouraged. Pooling of clinical experience is important for it is from clinical questions that research initiatives grow. For example, many therapists would say, from their own experience, that early intensive help for language-disordered children is important for good progress. However, to date, there is very little evidence to support this view (Hutt, 1986; Urwin, Cook and Kelly, 1988). If we wish to move towards establishing evidence to support, or deny, this view, we will need to consider more formal research procedures (see Chapter 8).

Other Ways of Working with Language-disordered Children

The speech therapist's task is not easy to define. Each of us will have a formal job description, but the way in which we carry it out will vary and, to a large extent, be determined by personal decisions and experience. The job is often quite large, involving a number of schools, clinics, nurseries and several groups of staff to work with. Not all the therapist's time will be spent in face-to-face contact with a language-disordered child. Although a certain amount of time will need to be devoted to being an advisor or carrying out administrative tasks, getting the balance right can be quite a headache. Management policy might describe a flexible approach to the provision of care for these children, but in reality that may simply mean trying to reduce the length of the waiting list.

Traditional patterns of treatment were often regular, such as once weekly, and extensive, over several years, until the problem seemed to have resolved. Few therapists would have the time to take such an approach now even if it still seemed the most sensible. The trend in treatment patterns appears to be towards a much more goal-oriented progamme in which specific needs are worked on in 'blocks' of several weeks or months which then continue in a cyclic pattern depending on the needs of the children concerned. To set up a timetable that is both flexible and effective within a clinical environment is like spinning plates: it is necessary to keep control of several factors at any one time. For example, let us suppose the task is to set up a timetable for two sessions per week to provide group work for language-disordered children in nurseries or schools from a community clinic base. The following steps will be required:

1. Contact up to two local schools or nurseries where there is a current need for more intensive and specific language work and where the language-disordered children are already known.
2. Explain why these venues have been chosen. This may be a short-term need and, if the children leave, the service will need to be reallocated. Emphasise which group of children the service is aimed at, e.g. children aged 4–5 years with severe phonological problems. Others should continue to be referred in the usual way but their needs will have to be met differently, perhaps in another course.
3. Discuss the proposed format of the course with the other staff as appropriate. In effect, take out a contract with them to provide this specific service. This should include how often the group(s) will run, which children will attend, whether other staff will take part etc.
4. Set up the timetable for the groups: for example half a term for initial observations, planning, training and liaisons. This is followed by half a term in nursery class A, then time for evaluation and planning out of term time, followed by half a term in class B followed by evaluation and planning etc. Where it is not possible to work within the nursery or school similar plan could be proposed within the clinic.

If the clinician chooses this approach, initially the work load is heavy, but once the system begins to get under way, it is fairly straightforward to adjust and move on to the next group. Regular and consistent contact with staff will increase awareness about language disorder, although it is important to remember that staff may change and new staff will need further training. There is no right answer to the planning of patterns of therapy for language-disordered children. However, provided the children's needs are kept central when proposing a system or programme, a flexible approach is to be encouraged where it maximises staff expertise and resources.

Chapter 8
Research: Methods and Issues

Summary

Several methods appropriate to clinical research with language-impaired children are discussed including longitudinal studies, case descriptions and single case designs. The importance of supervision is emphasised with regard to research.

We all have our prejudices about research: some of us are very keen on the idea and others never see themselves as being involved. As with most prejudices, our negative feelings about research are probably largely a result of ignorance and doubt. Most students of speech therapy, psychology or medicine are expected to produce a piece of original work, loosely termed a 'project' or 'dissertation', that is relevant to their future clinical practice. However, it is not our intention to suggest that the already over-worked clinician should take on the additional role of researcher. Some aspects of the investigation of language impairment will require full-time research fellowships. This does not mean that therapists in clinical practice do not need to be aware of research methodology; they may find themselves better equipped to be involved in clinical research trials. It is true that those in clinical work may find themselves at an initial disadvantage when planning research, because the basic requirements of experimental research do not seem to equate straight away with the clinical situation.

Experimental research	vs	*Clinical research*
Careful specification of independent variables		Experimental conditions not well specified
Dependent measures must be objective and replicable		Dependent measures used to evaluate performance usually not objective

170

However, a broader view of the clinician's aims and strategies reveals much common ground between these two positions. As Compton (1976) comments, in relation to a sound production task:

> In the process of selecting the specific key sounds to include in therapy, we arc formulating our working hypothesis of the most effective route to follow in correcting a child's speech; the effects of therapy upon the child's speech constitutes a test of these hypotheses. With each child, we are conducting an experiment, the result of which allows us to further refine our hypotheses and thereby improve the effectiveness of therapy. In this sense the dichotomy between therapy and research is totally without foundation.

We support Compton's affirmation that every clinical situation is a potential research field. The clinician is always generating hypotheses, collecting data and analysing them. Yet very few of these hypotheses are formalised, and few of the data are analysed or discussed publicly. Whilst we are not suggesting that it is appropriate for every clinical situation to be treated in this way, the furthering of our knowledge of language impairment does require more involvement in the research process. In order to be better equipped to take part in this process we need to consider three main areas: (1) the questions we should ask, (2) the method(s) that could answer the question(s) and (3) how to 'do' research.

What Questions should we ask?

As previously discussed in Chapter 3, when considering the process of differential diagnosis, the main questions facing the clinician are:

1. How severe is the problem now?
2. Will intervention help and if so what?
3. What is the prognosis?

These questions are a reasonable place to start and other questions are bound to evolve from them. It is quite usual to find that there are too many questions, or the questions are really too big to answer in their present form.

Questions about the severity of the presenting problem, or the features of the condition, are very relevant in language impairment. Some objective measures which evaluate the severity and describe the features of children's language problems do exist (see Chapter 2 under 'Formal and informal assessment'). Some of these are now being more vigorously applied to the diagnosis of language impairment (see Chapter 3 for a discussion of an expert system). However, this is a continually growing area; new instruments of assessment continue to be developed for specific population groups. Commonly these grow from a descriptive base, such as the Checklist of Pragmatic Skills of Dewart and Summers (1988), through a stage in which agreed measures are assigned to descriptions (e.g. Gerard's (1986) Checklist of Communicative Competence) to a stage where descriptions and objective measures can be related (this is the aim of the Paediatric Oral Skills Checklist*).

Questions about the efficacy of intervention strategies have become a contentious area in recent years. The question 'Does speech therapy work?' is one of the enormous ones, but it does not mean that smaller, more carefully defined versions of this question should not be considered. A rewording of the question may become: 'What is the effect of X in this situation, with this population/group/client'. Questions of this type commonly fill whole hosts of research journals.

Questions about prognosis are usually of prime concern to parents and carers, and are important to our planning for the future needs of our client group(s). Yet we have rarely documented the course of language problems or described their residual effects in sufficient detail for such information to be available. Some studies may overlap a number of questions. Lees's (1989) study of acquired childhood aphasia set out to document the course and prognosis of the condition, and use objective tests to measure the severity of the aphasia during this time (see Chapter 9 for further discussion). French (1989) used a hierarchically organised sound matching task with a small group of children with severe comprehension problems to see if the children's progress with this type of intervention could be used as a measure of the severity of their problem. By constructing simple tasks which moved through listening, matching sounds to objects, matching sounds to pictures and then matching new sounds, she was able to show that this group of four children could be taught in a structured situation but what they learned was not generalised to the new material.

When focusing on a question around which to generate a hypothesis for clinical research, the main considerations need to be the size of the question, its scope and manageability, and the relevance of the question to clinical practice. Most of all is it a question that the researcher really wants to answer?

What Method(s) would answer the Question(s)?

Different professional groups have generally evolved a tendency to adopt particular research methods to answer the questions posed in their clinical situation. Some of these research methods have been used in clinical

---

* Contact Janet Lees at the Department of Clinical Genetics, St George's Hospital Medical School, London for information about this checklist

research with language-disordered children. Others have not been tried with this population specifically, but have been used in other areas of research in communication disorders. This overview is brief and not intended to be a comprehensive evaluation of these methodologies. Rather it is intended to introduce clinicians to the range of possibilities available. Anyone intending to begin serious clinical research is advised to seek further specific advice.

Longitudinal studies

The practice of selecting a group of children on the basis of some specific criteria, determining the timespan over which the group will be studied and then sampling a particular behaviour at certain times during the study is a common method used for determining the natural history of many developmental disorders in childhood. It forms the basis of studies of developmental language problems such as those of Bishop and Edmundson (1987) and of acquired ones like Lees (1989). Whilst it might seem simple enough to set up, there are a number of preliminary considerations. The first concerns the selection of the group. If the object of the study is to discern trends in the evolution of behaviour which can be generalised to other groups of children, the sample size will be important. Statistically significant trends are less likely to appear in a small group unless they are particularly striking. However, if a large group is recruited, other difficulties arise. First, the number of hours required to see all the subjects is increased along with the time taken to analyse the data. A further consideration with a longitudinal study will be the number of subjects who become lost to follow-up for various reasons (move away, withdraw consent etc.).

The criteria on which the children are selected will depend on the question to be answered. If a developmental pattern is being investigated, then the most important criterion will be that the child is at the right age or developmental level to enter the study. The more critieria that are considered to be significant to the selection of the children, the harder it will be to recruit subjects. Similarly the timespan of the study may influence how many children are lost to follow-up, with it being more difficult to keep track of large groups of children over several years unless a central register is used. The timespan will also influence the way in which the study is conducted – one major worker or a succession of several for the various stages. The time intervals at which the behaviour is sampled will depend to some extent on what is already known about the disorder and the hypothesis to be tested. For example, Bishop and Edmundson (1987) set up their study to consider the hypothesis of maturational lag as an explanation for delay in language development. Thus they took a sizeable sample of children in order to discern any signifcant trend. They sampled a range of language abilities, using formal tests, and other aspects of development to see how these evolved together. The study ended in the middle of childhood after the period thought to be significant for language development (up to 5 years of age). Some variables could not be controlled for within the study, for example amount of speech therapy the children had received. Thus they were unable to draw any conclusions about the significance of this factor in the outcome, either for individuals or the group. The advantage of a longitudinal study is that, with careful planning, sampling can be spread out or occur in blocks depending on the researchers' preference. Armed with information about natural history we are in a better position to consider the appropriate timing of therapy or measure the effect of intervention.

Case descriptions:

A case description is just that – a description of a case. This method of reporting clinical observations is commonly used in many branches of medicine, including child development, clinical genetics and psychiatry. The range of human behaviour is very wide and previously unreported phenomena do continue to appear from time to time. Equally, new techniques of management may be reported in descriptive terms before they can be reported to have achieved statistically significant results. With these points in mind, the case description would appear to be a useful method of reporting that could be used in speech and language pathology. It has been used to define syndromes like the Landau–Kleffner syndrome (Landau and Kleffner, 1957).

To prepare a case description, the fullest possible information about the child needs to be available. Because this method makes no attempt to control for variables, it is important to document what all the possible variables in each case might be. A full history of the child should be given, including the family history. When describing the particular behaviour of interest, care should be taken to make this as clear as possible. The use of objective measures will be important in achieving this, because it will help other workers to identify similarities in other children. Where possible a profile of indentifying features should be included. Subjective language can form a part of case descriptions, but should be relevant and not extraneous. Most case descriptions form the initial basis for indentifying a condition or behaviour, or for describing a possible management strategy so that it can be further defined, evaluated or tested through a more stringent procedure.

It is important to remember the limitations of the method. First, the clarity of the description may be open to a range of interpretations. Secondly, where a response to treatment is described, it must be remembered that this has not been validated against controls. It may be that such a response was just a feature of the natural history of the condition and not related to treatment. Without control measures, this cannot be determined; however, this is still a useful place to begin clinical research with language-disordered children. The literature contains too few objective descriptions of this type and even fewer attempts to describe response to treatment. Jarvis's (1989) case description of a child with a phonological disorder is a good example of this method. She gives a clear picture of the child's presenting problem and a logical discussion of the reasoning behind the choice of therapeutic approach (in this case, metaphon therapy). The child's responses are detailed over time and the results are also presented on a graph. There is no case-control element to the study, but the clinician can decide, from the information provided, if he or she has a child like this with whom this approach might be feasible. However, a more stringent test of the effectiveness of metaphon therapy would require a different methodology.

Single case designs

These may provide possible alternatives which include some control of the variables needed to evaluate the effectiveness of language therapy in children. The basic premise underlying the various types in this group is that the subject acts as his or her own control. Thus periods of treatment are placed in sequence with periods of non-treatment, and the progress made under these different conditions is evaluated to see if the progress with treatment was significantly better than the progress without treatment. The advantage of this method is that the number of cases involved at any time can be as small as one. It is possible to use a single case design within a group. In such a situation, each child continues to act as her or his own control but the same therapy is delivered to more than one child. The major disadvantage of this method is the number of assessments that are required during the course of a study to demonstrate and then reconfirm any treatment effect. It also requires that the therapy programme is carefully specified and specifically targeted.

Basically, the methodology requires a pre-treatment period in which the child is assessed or observed, and a baseline method of the behaviour under consideration is established. Once the baseline is established, the treatment can be introduced, after which the behaviour is measured again and any change from the baseline documented. It is usual, in the more stringent studies, to revert to a non-treatment condition to observe whether the behaviour changes again, after which a further treatment period can be introduced and any further changes documented. This is a so-called ABAB design where A stands for non-treatment and B stands for the treatment period. Variations on this theme include a multiple baseline method in which several different behaviours can be measured in the initial non-treatment period, followed by the introduction of a specific treatment aimed at one of the behaviours. After the first period or treatment, the reassessment in the non-treatment period establishes any change in treated or non-treated behaviour. A further period of treatment, perhaps targeted at a different behaviour, followed by a further period of observation can be useful in establishing whether treatment effects are specific (progress occurs in the treated behaviour only) or generalised (progress occurs in both treated and untreated behaviours). When using single case designs in the treatment of language-disordered children, it is important to remember that they do take quite a lot of time to set up and that the results are specific to the child. The shifting baseline of child development may influence the treatment and non-treatment periods, but it may be difficult to say in exactly what way this happens. For a fuller discussion of setting up such a study the reader is referred to Kratochwill (1978) and Kazdin (1982), both of whom deal with these subjects from a clinical perspective.

Other methodologies

A more traditional methodology used in medical research, but which has been found to be rather limiting in speech and language research with adult subjects, is the randomised control trial. In such studies, it is usual to have a large group of subjects and allocate them at random to a number of different experimental and control conditions. The progress made under each condition for the group as a whole is then averaged out and the significance of the result calculated. The major problem with this methodology for language-disordered children is that speech therapy is not usually (if ever) allocated on a random basis. Children are selected for therapy on the basis of a wide range of criteria such as age, developmental level, attention level, attention span, presenting disorder, social and group skills, motivation, auditory verbal memory, verbal comprehension skills etc. Some of these factors could be controlled for, but the larger the number of controlled variables the harder it is to recruit children to the study. A random allocation of children suggests that the experimenter expects the overall effects of therapy to be similar in terms of timing of progress and overall improvement. One thing that is quite clear about the population of language-disordered children is that the range is so wide and individual development so varied that such a simplistic notion is not likely to be upheld. Such a study would probably result in a predictably non-significant result. Pring (1987) questions the need to use this type of methodology to evaluate aphasia therapy with adults, due to the uncertainty about what aphasia therapy is. It is not like a measured dose of medicine. Given the state of discussion about language therapy with children and the problem of the shifting baseline of child development, it would seem to be no more appropriate for this group either.

Eastwood (1986) has proposed that qualitative research, as used in a number of the social sciences including anthropology, would be a useful methodology for speech and language research. She defines the main principles of qualitative research as:

1. An initial investigation of the situation in which the researcher does not make reference to hypothesis or theory but confines his or her attention to accurate observation. This is sometimes referred to as a 'fishing expedition'.
2. The value of the researcher's subjective view point is recognised as being equal to objective measurement. The biases which any research contributes by including a subjective view must be clarified but are not discarded.
3. The research is carried out in a specific situation or setting and is specific to that location.
4. The researcher seeks to clarify the behaviour which is studied by suggesting explanations for its occurrence. In this respect he or she draws on hypothesis and theories for explanation for what has been observed.

Qualitative research, therefore, has four principal components: observation, description, self-reflection and interpretation. This would appear to neatly summarise the process adopted by a clinician in the treatment of a language-impaired child, and would suggest that the concept of qualitative research is worth further investigation for those seeking to understand the therapeutic process.

How to do Research

For the clinician seriously intent on entering the research field, some of the most important personal considerations will be motivation and organisational skills. Many questions may arise in clinical practice; some will surface many times and stimulate greater interest. It is of the greatest importance to have an interesting and relevant question. Because of the amount of time and effort which the researcher will invest in any study, it is essential to be committed fully to the question under consideration. Once set on finding an answer to a question, the researcher should discuss the practical aspects of the decision with a colleague or member of an academic department who already has research experience and who can therefore help to spot the pitfalls and plan a course of action. For all types of studies, the major considerations will be finance and time which clearly influence each other. There is no point in trying to do complex research without being able to devote sufficient time to it – such a course is just frustrating. Equally, finance will be required either to free time and/or provide extra staff or equipment. Applying for a research grant is usually the first step. A joint application with an already experienced colleague, or an application to work within a larger study, can be a good starting point.

Supervision is fundamentally important to the success of the study. Specific time for supervision needs to be set aside at the planning stage. The choice of supervisor is important but the characteristics of a good supervisor are very subjective. In the first place it needs to be someone the researcher can work in partnership with, because this will be a mutual learning experience. Clearly it needs to be someone with a good working knowledge of the subject. Although there may be one formal supervisor, the support of other colleagues will be important for different parts of the study. You will want to discuss your findings widely and some may have more specific experience to contribute, particularly when it comes to statistical analysis.

A literature search will form the introduction to the study and sharpen the questions at issue. Most large academic libraries can arrange for a computer literature search for a fee. Many ideas and further questions will probably come to mind for consideration and discussion once data collection is underway. The final presentation of the study in written or verbal form will be very satisfying and is quite likely to be accompanied by the discovery of further questions which will form the basis of the next study.

Not everyone will want to get involved in a large study, but many will be interested in a smaller, and more manageable, part. This may involve collecting data in a particular way over a specific period or identifying possible subjects for inclusion in someone else's study. Where children in the therapist's care are a part of a study, there is no need to find this intimidating in the management of the case. Those involved in language research may be looking for answers, but few would claim to have found them all yet. Nor are they likely to be in any sense unwilling to discuss and share preliminary findings or views. Personal experience suggests that it is through opportunities to discuss the study with co-workers that further ideas and questions are generated. Clinical observations make an important contribution to developing models and research priorities for language-disordered children.

Chapter 9
Acquired Childhood Aphasia

Summary

Children who present with acquired language problems are discussed from a clinical perspective and with reference to a recent longitudinal study. A procedure for the assessment of these children is presented. The different problems of those with head injury, unilateral cerebral lesion and the Landau–Kleffner syndrome are discussed. The question of recovery from acquired aphasia in childhood is also addressed.

The majority of generalist paediatric speech therapists will rarely see a child with acquired aphasia, although some specialists, particularly those working in children's hospitals, will be more familiar with this group of language-impaired children. Robinson (1987) reported two series of children: one from a child development centre and one from a school for speech and language-disordered children. Acquired language problems only accounted for between 4% and 7% of the children in these two groups. Whilst the numbers of children with acquired language problems may be smaller than those with developmental ones, the range of causes of loss or deterioration of language in childhood is wide. In all of them there is neurological evidence to suggest cerebral dysfunction. This includes focal and diffuse cerebral injury as well as acute or chronic disease processes and transient or fluctuating conditions. It may be the result of trauma or related to the presence of ongoing epileptic activity. Table 9.1 summarises the causes of loss or deterioration of language in childhood.

Some clinical differences may be observed in the presenting features and the management priorities. Most of the research on this population has tended to consider three groups: language problems related to head injury in childhood, aphasia secondary to unilateral cerebral lesions and aphasia with convulsive disorder, particularly the Landau–Kleffner syndrome. These will be discussed separately but first the clinical features of acquired childhood aphasia (ACA) need to be considered together with suitable assessment procedures.

Table 9.1   Causes of loss or deterioration of language in childhood

Head injury: open or closed
   Diffuse and bilateral damage may be combined with additional focal damage

   Additional problems may include motor, cognitive and sensory deficits, so
   influencing rehabilitation needs

   Epilepsy may be a sequela

   Where initial aphasia is very severe and persists for more than 6 months,
   prognosis for complete recovery is poor

   In young children, later acquisition of written language may be impaired

Unilateral cerebrovascular lesions
   Damage is essentially focal

   Visual field defects and hemiplegia may also occur

   Epilepsy may be a sequela

   Even when initial aphasia is severe a return to within −2 s.d. for verbal
   comprehension score within 6 months of onset is usually indicative of a good
   prognosis

Cerebral infections
   Meningitis and encephalitis
      Usually diffuse effect, and additional motor, cognitive and sensory deficits
      are common in severe cases

   Cerebral abscess
      Essentially a focal effect, probably to temporal or frontal lobes
      Where the damage is purely cortical the aphasia is usually only moderate to
      mild

Convulsive aphasia
   Aphasia may occur as a consequence of convulsive status, as a post-ictal
   phenomenon, or as a feature of minor epileptic status

   Other learning problems may also occur in association, particularly after long
   and repeated convulsive status

   Language disturbance may be fleeting, short term (less than 24 hours), more
   long term or fluctuating

Table 9.1 (*contd*)

Landau–Kleffner syndrome

    May be preceded or followed by epilepsy but one-third of cases never have epilepsy

    Major feature of language is a severe receptive aphasia

    Language comprehension may deteriorate over a long period. Where this shows little recovery over first 6 months, the prognosis is poor

    Loss of language comprehension may be acute, sometimes in association with another illness. Where recovery is good in first 3 months (to within -2 s.d.) prognosis is good

    Language comprehension may fluctuate in association with temporal lobe EEG abnormalities. Where this can be controlled by anticonvulsants, prognosis is moderate to good

Other syndromes

    Late-onset autism

        A pervasive developmental disorder of the autistic type which is preceded by a period of normal development

        Loss of social and communication skills are the major signs. Severe receptive language disorder is common. There may be an accompanying deterioration in other cognitive skills

    Rett's syndrome

        Developmental disorder in which motor and cognitive skills are lost between 6 and 12 months of age

        All known cases are girls

        Other clinical signs include: inappropriate social interaction, slowing of head growth, severe communication difficulties, abnormal oral movements

Other disintegrative disorders of childhood

    The term 'pervasive developmental disorders' includes a group of acquired, late-onset or otherwise deteriorating conditions which affect cognitive, social and language skills but which are as yet poorly identified, in terms of aetiology, symptomatology and prognosis

    In general, those in which the greatest range of skills is lost, in which severe epilepsy occurs and in which little progress is made in the first 6 months after onset are associated with a poor prognosis

Assessment of Acquired Childhood Aphasia

As previously discussed, speech therapy intervention must begin with appropriate assessment and diagnosis (see Chapters 2 and 3). However, this is often not so straightforward for the child with ACA for the following reasons:

1. The complex association of motor, cognitive, perceptual, emotional and communication problems which can arise from brain injury, both localised and diffuse.
2. The fact that very little formal assessment material is available specifically for these children.
3. The changing nature of the deficits both for those recovering very quickly and for those making little progress.
4. The uncommon nature of the problem and the relative inexperience in this specialised area.

Reassessment is clearly important in measuring recovery. As each individual child's response to brain injury will vary, the only way to know what stage the child is at and how to establish the next goal for intervention is to use an appropriate protocol. This is particularly pertinent in the following circumstances:

1. Where the situation is changing rapidly, i.e. in the initial recovery period, as it is important that intervention keeps up with this.
2. Where the situation is rather static, i.e. in the later stages of recovery, to see where the specific deficits are.
3. Where therapy is being given, to evaluate its effect and redirect goals as necessary.
4. Where the child is said to have 'recovered' but it still experiencing difficulty at school, to see if any residual problems are being overlooked.

It is important to establish a comprehensive profile of the child's speeech and language over time. Whilst informal observations will be important, particularly in acute stages, formal measures will be an advantage when making peer group comparisons and measuring progress. In order to choose the most appropriate test instruments to establish this profile, the clinician needs to be aware of the main types of language difficulties encountered in acquired language disorders in childhood. These are:

1. Auditory—verbal comprehension problems: difficulty understanding spoken language. Hecaen (1976) described this in about one-third of his cases.
2. Word-finding problems: difficulty recalling specific words. Generally the most prominent feature of ACA.

3. Jargon aphasia: incomprehensible expressive language. Van Dongen, Loonen and Van Dongen (1985) described three cases.
4. Semantic and phonemic paraphasias: naming errors which show a semantic or phonemic relationship to the target word. Van Hout, Evrard and Lyon (1985) described a series of these.
5. Perseveration: persistent, undifferentiated error responses. Described in a small number of brain-injured children (Lees, 1989).

Informal assessment and screening procedures, such as the Children's Aphasia Screening Test (Whurr and Evans, 1986) may be useful in the initial stages. However, the mildly or moderately aphasic child soon reaches the ceiling on such tests, and they rarely provide a detailed enough profile for long-term use in the severely aphasic child. The choice of formal assessment will depend on the stage of recovery the child is at and the level of cooperation. It should be emphasised that developmental assessments, such as the Reynell Development Language Scales (Reynell, 1977), are rarely able to describe the specific difficulties of this group. A battery of tests which establish a profile of abilities is recommended from clinical and research experience (Lees, 1989). This includes the following tests.

A test for auditory–verbal comprehension

The Test for Reception of Grammar (Bishop, 1983) is the preferred test. It has comprehension norms, good presentation which can also be used with motor-impaired children (by eye pointing if necessary) and it is reliable for reassessment purposes in a changing situation.

A test of confrontational naming

There are several useful tests depending on the age of the child: these include the Word Finding Vocabulary Test (Renfrew, 1972c) and the Test of Word Finding (German, 1986). The latter is particularly useful in providing a framework for analysing the types of cues the child uses to aid word finding (German, 1989). The Graded Naming Test (McKenna and Warrington, 1983) can be used with teenagers. Some preliminary norms are available (Lees, 1989).

A comparison with association naming

If the Test for Word Finding (German, 1986) is used, then this is a subsection of this test. Otherwise, the Auditory Association subtest of the Illinois Test of Psycholinguistic Abilities (ITPA) is quite useful (Kirk, McCarthy and Kirk, 1968).

A sample of expressive language

It may be necessary to use a technique like 'story telling' to elicit this where the child is rather reticent (not uncommon after ACA).

Other investigations

These may include short-term memory, using sentence repetition or word lists, or other aspects of auditory processing including the internal manipulation of phonemes in auditory discrimination tests or the production of rhyming or alliterative words, singly or in lists.

Head Injury

The largest group of children with acquired language problems comprises those who suffer head injuries of various severities. The recovery of their speech and language abilities has considerable implications for the educational placement, social integration, family and peer relationships, and all aspects of the child's future development. However, there is little specific provision for the rehabilitation of head-injured children. Few speech therapists in the UK specialise in this work. This means that children are often seen in establishments poorly suited to their individual needs. These are not the only problems. Few previous studies of this group have used adequate investigations of language to establish either the features of acquired language problems in detail, the course of recovery or the outcome. Speech therapists seeing these children as a part of a general paediatric caseload, within a school for physically handicapped children or even in a general hospital frequently ask similar questions in an attempt to understand the complex management problems they present.

Since the early 1980s the number of children referred with acquired language problems after head injury has increased. This seems to be due to two factors: first, better intensive care facilities, including the use of intracranial pressure monitoring, leading to more child survivors of severe head injuries and, secondly, the introduction of the 1981 Education Act, which makes provision for the assessment of children with special educational needs. As we shall see, the residual language problems after head injury in childhood can cover a wide range and require comprehensive assessment if they are to be suitably managed.

According to research mentioned by Ewing-Cobbs et al. (1985), head injury is the most common cause of death in children. They emphasised the size of the population, the mechanisms of trauma and the response of the injured brain. Although diffuse cerebral injury at impact is the major effect, other forces of acceleration, shearing and stretching occur, resulting in wide-spread injury to the cerebral tissues. This damage is sometimes shown up by advanced radiographic techniques, such as magnetic resonance imaging. Few studies have documented the recovery of cognitive and language skills in head-injured children. The resolution of acute neurology is only a small measure of recovery in children who have sustained complex brain injury. Long-term neuropsychological deficits are more likely to affect the quality of life, the return to the former community and progress within school.

In order to establish the short-term needs of these children, Ewing-Cobbs et al. (1985) looked at the language function of a group of children 5 months after complex head injury. They found aphasic language problems in less than 10% of the sample and concluded that language difficulties after paediatric head injury were 'non-specific in nature, and did not vary consistently with the type of cerebral involvement' (p. 104). The need for long-term follow-up was also emphasised, particularly as it had been suggested that problems in the later acquisition of language skills, such as reading, may be delayed following head injury in children.

There is little consensus about the length of follow-up time which constitutes a long-term study. Jordan, Ozanne and Murdoch (1988) examined a group of 20 children aged 8–16 years who had sustained complex head injury at least 12 months previously. They found language test scores of the head-injured group to be significantly lower than the control group. The performance of both groups on the Frenchay Dysarthria Test (Enderby, 1983) was well within the normal range, so they do not appear to have had motor speech problems, which can complicate the clinical presentation after head injury in childhood. They concluded that it was important to include both long- and short-term monitoring of language in this group.

Concern about intellectual performance, scholastic achievement and particularly the long-term effect on reading skills, formed the basis of the study by Chadwick et al. (1981) of 97 children, who were at least 2 years post head injury. A wide range of psychological tests and tests of scholastic achievement tended to show a greater impairment following left hemisphere lesions. This tendency was most marked in children under 5 years of age at the time of injury. Although they agree that this needs further study, they state that it could mean that 'brain injury is more likely to impair the acquisition of new skills than to cause the loss of well established old skills' (p. 134). General intellectual impairment was found to be significantly associated with the overall severity of the original trauma.

What is the evolution of speech and language difficulty after head injury in childhood?

The recovery of head-injured children can be considered in three stages; the length of the stages is variable and probably depends on the severity of the injury.

The acute period

This is the period from emergency admission to the re-establishment of the stable conscious state; the trauma team will be at its most active. Neurosurgery, various investigations and intensive care monitoring may all be a necessary part of the management. If there is a long period of unconsciousness when the child is stable, therapists may become involved in coma stimulation therapies. Physiotherapists concentrate on the possible range of movements and the prevention of deforming contractures. Speech therapists may be involved in appropriate auditory stimulation, which can include tapes of well-known sounds and voices, as well as the establishment of a consistent pattern of greetings and instructions to accompany regular nursing care. Coma stimulation may involve other senses, including touch, smell and taste, which may be a basic prerequisite to re-establishing communication. A small number of children may return to consciousness but make no further progress; this is described as a 'persistent vegetative state'.

A *period of consistent recovery*

This period may be very short in the mildly or moderately injured child or may last for several years in a more severely injured child. It is a time for therapy and educational imput to maximise recovery. Thorough and ongoing assessment needs to be carried out, and goal-oriented treatment programmes used to aim towards functional rehabilitation. Where progress through this period is fast, the child may appear to regain quickly the normal range on a number of skills. This does not mean, however, that more long-term difficulties may not develop later, particularly when the child returns to school.

Plateauing of recovery and long-term residual deficits

The time it takes for the child to reach this stage will again depend on the severity of the injury. Only consistent and comprehensive assessment will reveal whether progress is tailing off. Where there is a return to more or less normal previous levels, at least in some skills; long-term residual problems in others may be overlooked. Where there are multiple persisting deficits a consistent, specific and intensive approach to treatment is probably necessary.

At all stages of recovery an emphasis must be placed on the integrated multidisciplinary working of the therapy, medical, social and educational services for the benefit of the individual child and the family. These children's problems are too complex for an individual professional to 'solve' alone. The team may require a team leader or key worker, and this is often best done by a therapist who has knowledge of the roles of the other team members, rather than by a medical consultant as in the more traditional models.

The management of speech and language problems in the head-injured child

When a profile of language skills has been obtained, it can be used to set treatment goals and monitor progress. The graphs (see Figures 9.1 and 9.2) shown for Cases 19 and 20 demonstrate one method of monitoring the child's progress. They allow the clinician to see how the child's performance compares with the normal range and what kind of progress towards the norm is being made. Followed up over time, such graphs show where the period of fastest recovery is, when the child's recovery starts to slow down and any mismatch that might develop between specific language functions. These considerations are helpful in determining the timing and specific focus of therapy.

In the very earliest stages of recovery, the head-injury child may have no communication at all, or only able to communicate non-verbally. It is not appropriate to leave a child with severe communication difficulties and the family without speech therapy support in the initial period of rapid recovery, even if the signs are that the child will get better. Both the child and the family will need informed and sensitive help to cope with communication difficulties which arise. Sometimes alternative or augmentative communication may be appropriate in the immediate post-trauma period to ease communication problems. However, it is not a straightforward matter of supplying a communication aid and leaving the child, family and other staff to get on with it. The following considerations are important:

1. The child's reaction to sudden loss of communication and other skills may be 'catastrophic'. After head injury in children a condition of post-traumatic mutism has been described. Levin et al. (1983) state that mutism is more common after head injury in children than in adults. They give an account of the recovery of a 12-year-old girl who was mute for 3 weeks post-trauma. It is not clear whether this is primarily related to the overall effect of the cerebral damage or if it is a psychological reaction to loss of function. The length of this period varies; Hecaen (1976) reports a range of up to 21 days. It may affect all communication modalities or be specifically related to the ability to use verbal language. The child may or may not be interested in using an alternative communication device during this time.
2. The family may insist on 'normality' of approach and equate alternative communication with the acceptance of handicap. The traumatic effect of the head injury is not only related to the injury to the child's brain.

The family too is 'injured' and reactions of grief and loss need to be worked through. Coming to terms with the effect of the injury is sometimes described by families as mourning for the child they have lost and getting to know the head-injured child as a new member of the family. This reaction probably relates to the considerable physical, cognitive and personality changes that can be the sequelae of severe head injury.

3. The associated motor, visual and perceptual problems may limit the choice of system or device. Whilst thay may not be insurmountable in the long term, such problems probably do require the experience of a multidisciplinary team. The provision of computer hardware, software and switches, in itself a complex area, will require the combined approach of an experienced multidisciplinary team. A number of national centres exist to advise about the provision of communication aids. However, in the short term, a less 'hi-tech' approach and the use of common sense may be the best answer.

4. Underlying language and cognitive problems may mean that, where complex instructions are required, the child cannot understand how to use the device. Non-verbal demonstration is probably the best answer to this problem. Some time spent just playing alongside the child and with the family, seeing if it fits their communication needs, is also essential.

5. The speed at which the problem changes may mean the device is only appropriate for a short time and needs frequent changing or adjustment, hence the importance of regular reviews.

With regard to these points, the following methods are recommended, particularly in the early stages of recovery.

Gestural support for communication

This may be introduced informally and later developed into a more formal system, perhaps within the framework of the Makaton vocabulary (Walker, 1980). Basic gestures/signs should be used consistently by all those working with the child, e.g. nurses, therapists, medical staff, teachers etc. It is usually helpful to ask the family to suggest the things they want to communicate to/with the child and where possible take up the child's own suggestions.

Child-specific communication boards

These should be as appropriate to the child as possible. Personal photographs are often a good idea to stimulate interest, add a real element of communicative intent, aid recall and help the family to become involved in the project. Although some ready-made boards are available a multipurpose Perspex board is often more adaptable in keeping up with the child's changing needs.

In the later stages of recovery, before any effective therapy programme can be implemented, the severity of the specific deficits should be carefully investigated. Then a deficit-specific approach which is regularly reviewed is recommended for a therapy programme for the following reasons:

1. It can be graded in a step-like manner, based on the child's strengths and needs, e.g. when working through the range of auditory processing difficulties, it is important to begin therapy in a distraction-free environment, as far as auditory interference is concerned, where the child functions well, working up through various situations which the child may encounter with less ease, including the sound situations found at home and school both formal and informal.

2. When teaching the rule-based systems of language, such as syntax, a structured approach is preferred. Both the Colour Pattern Scheme (Lea, 1980) and the Derbyshire Language Scheme (Knowles and Masidlover, 1982) are useful.

3. A consistent approach to the use of cueing to aid confrontational naming and word finding allows the child to generalise these skills more readily. Experience suggests that the child may pass through different stages at which different types of cues aid recall. Work in adult aphasia (Howard et al., 1985) suggests that different types of cues may be effective over different time periods. Clinical experience suggests that children may use different cues even within the normal population (Lees, 1989). Commonly, the cues used early in recovery are gestural, with verbal description and phonemic cues developing as later strategies.

4. The child can be encouraged to develop a capacity for the self-monitoring of errors. When this is related to specific deficits, it can be more readily generalised. For the long-term benefit of the brain-injured child, relearning a self-monitoring strategy is of the greatest importance, both for social independence and educational placement.

5. Long stretches of individual therapy in traditional treatment centres may not always be the most appropriate management for teenagers with long-standing problems. The therapist needs to be as flexible as possible when considering the place, timing and style of therapy offered and its effect on motivation.

Motor speech problems may complicate the presenting language difficulty. The differential diagnosis of dysphasia and dysarthria, whilst theoretically straightforward, may be less so in practice. Although our primary concern is language, some of the difficulties in managing motor speech problems should be briefly outlined. The problems are similar to those encountered when assessing the child's language. Very little specific assessment material is available. Two types of assessment predominate.

The use of adult material

In this respect the Frenchay Dysarthria Test (Enderby, 1983) is most commonly used by speech therapists expressing a preference. However, it is difficult to use this test successfully with children under 8 years of age.

The use of informal material

Most therapists use their own informal assessments. These should include assessment of head position and general posture (in conjunction with a physiotherapist), the presence or absence of oral reflexes, the control of respiration and phonation, observation and movement of the facial musculature, dentition, swallowing and the control of saliva. It is advisable to include videofluoroscopic examination of the swallowing mechanism where there is any doubt about its efficiency. The major problem in the use of informal assessments is in developing an objective scoring or recording scheme which allows the therapist to document the situation accurately, to allow for reliable reassessment measures. At present we know of no formal assessment procedure that fulfils these criteria. However, work in progress by Brindley et al. to produce a paediatric oral skills checklist* seeks to redress this deficit.

The problem of treatment is complicated by the fact that most head-injured children do not present with one 'pure' type of dysarthria. Usually the motor pattern is mixed and may include both upper and lower motor neurone signs. Most therapists initially become familiar with the assessment and treatment of oral motor problems in children through working with those with cerebral palsy. Although such experience is useful, the motor problems of head-injured children are different. This is not only because of the mixed neurology arising from the diffuse cerebral damage but also because of the acquired nature of the problem. The head-injured child, depending on the degree of recovery, has had a wealth of pre-traumatic experience. The way in which this is remembered by the child will vary, but must be a consideration when planning treatment. It is certainly different from the child with the congenital motor disorder who had no previous experience of 'normality'. The presence of other problems, particularly in language and cognition and possibly sensorimotor, may

---

* Brindley, C., Lees, J., Moffat, V., Crane, S. and Cave, D., work in progress on Paediatric Oral Skills Checklist (publication in 1991). Information can be obtained from J. Lees, Research SpeechTherapist, Department of Clinical Genetics, St George's Hospital Medical School, London.

make it difficult for the head-injured child to understand what is required during treatment. Models need to be clearly presented within a structured framework. Frequent repetition of the desired target is also required in order to accommodate these difficulties and the variable attention span which may also be a feature.

Problems with written language may appear to be the most persistent language deficits after head injury in children. In this respect age of injury does not appear to be a determining factor in prognosis. Ewing-Cobbs et al. (1985) reported that head-injured children demonstrated greater difficulty with written language tests than head-injured adolescents, regardless of the severity of the injury. The few studies of written language problems in this population have failed to establish the level at which the processing of language breaks down. Also they have not outlined the strategies used by head-injured children to overcome reading and spelling problems. These are two important considerations when therapists and teachers seek to plan remedial programmes.

When seeing a head-injured child with reading and spelling problems, it is important to carry out a thorough language assessment to confirm that other difficulties really do not exist. Children referred with persistent spelling problems frequently also have high level, auditory comprehension problems, auditory discrimination problems and other difficulties with the discrimination and manipulation of phonemes, as well as word-finding problems, both general and specific. These high level language problems may have been difficult to be objective about in practice and so have been overlooked. It is also important to make a thorough investigation of reading and spelling strategies used by the child. Most children do develop strategies for overcoming current difficulties (even if it is a negative strategy such as 'don't know'). Working with the child will reveal which route is functional for the transposition of phonemes to graphemes (i.e. is the strategy predominantly based on visual memory, or is it phonetic?), what knowledge of errors the child has and what self-correction strategies, if any, are employed. It may be difficult to establish pre-trauma levels of language competence but it is important to look to see if there is any evidence of a family history of spelling difficulty or language problems. Clinical folklore abounds with stories about the numbers of head-injured children who were not very competent language users before injury. This should not be taken as an indication that the child would have had some reading and writing difficulties anyway, and that therefore nothing needs to be done. The combined effects of early developmental difficulty and further brain injury are likely to cause long-term problems and each child's needs must be individually assessed. The management of written language difficulties is best approached jointly, by speech therapist and teacher, if an appropriate remedial programme is to be implemented which is aimed at the child's educational needs and future language competence.

A comparison of the recovery of speech and language in two head-injured children

It is not possible in two cases to show the whole range of speech and language problems which might be encountered in this population. The two presented here are similar in age, but differ in terms of presenting symptoms, management and prognosis. An account of the medical background is given and then a discussion of the presenting problems, what was revealed by assessment and some of the residual difficulties.

Case 19

A girl with a normal developmental history was involved in a road traffic accident at the age of 12 years in which she sustained multiple injuries. She was admitted in an unconscious state with a severe head injury, ruptured spleen and haemorrhage, pneumothorax and chest injury, and fractures of the right clavicle and ankle (Glasgow Coma Score 5). A CT scan was reported to show subarachnoid blood over the right cerebellar hemisphere, within the vermis and the fourth ventricle, and the right lateral ventricle. There were two dissociated intracerebral bleeds and virtually no oedema. This was described as a general cerebral contusion. A repeat scan 24 hours later, prompted by her deteriorating condition, was unchanged. However, another scan 7 days later suggested that the haematomas were less desnse, although there was little change in the size of the ventricles.

She was nursed in intensive care for 4 weeks, during the first week of which she was critically ill. Ultrasonic angiography at this stage showed no evidence of occlusion of the extracranial carotid arteries and middle cerebral artery flow was detected to be similar bilaterally. However, there was a suggestion of increased and turbulent flow in the left jugular and possible obstruction in the right jugular. Once she was out of the critical care stage, she had evidence of a very severe motor disorder with spasticity in the right limbs and extrapyramidal signs on the left side including tremor.

Six weeks post-trauma she began to show some awareness of her surroundings and 10 weeks postinjury she was responding to being spoken to. She still had a profound motor disorder and a receptive and expressive dysphasia. Twelve weeks postinjury she was making steady progress and marked improvements were noted: she was responsive, cooperative, cheerful and talking. There had been a great improvement in motor function; the right side was still worse than the left, but she had reasonable hand function on both sides, could sit independently and walk with support. She continued to make excellent progress from her severe head injury and was discharged to a weekly boarding placement for rehabilitation where she gained sufficient mobility to walk independently. She continued to make good progress with language and learning, within this structured environment. Both education and therapy were well integrated, goal oriented and directed to specific deficits. Two years post-trauma she was transferred to another school for children with physical difficulties nearer her home, with only moderate residual motor problems and a slight dysarthria. Figure 9.1 shows her progress over the 2-year recovery period.

Assessment of naming difficulties on the Word Finding Vocabulary Test shows the types and range of naming errors early

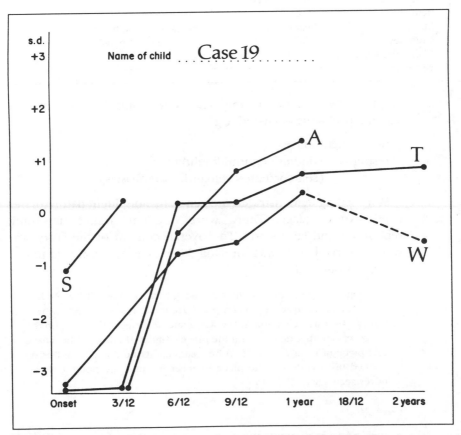

Figure 9.1   Language profile graph of Case 19. T = TROG; A = auditory association; S = sentence repetition; W = word finding

Table 9.2   Initial assessment of Case 19 2 months post-trauma

Item	Response	Error types
Cup	Cup	
Table	Table	
Boat	Sink	Semantic paraphasia
Tree	Glass	Semantic paraphasia
Key	Key	
Knife	Knife	
Window	Table	Semantic paraphasia
Finger	Finger	
Duck	Duck	
Snake	Table	Perseveration
Basket	Table	Perseveration
Saw	Knife	Semantic paraphasia
Pear	Pear	
Clown	Dog	Semantic paraphasia
Case	(No response)	
Bear	Dog	Perseveration
Moon	Pear	Semantic paraphasia
Chimney	Chair	Semantic paraphasia
(Test discontinued)		

in the recovery period (Table 9.2). Nine months post-onset some naming problems persisted, e.g.

item – lighthouse
response – windmill/lightmill/lighthouse
                    (self-corrected semantic paraphasias)

Story telling demonstrated the generally non-fluent nature of her expressive language. There were frequent hesitations, some repetitions and false starts. The overall content of the story was well preserved. This was the Dog Story (see Appendix II) told 6 months post-onset:

> The dog had a piece of meat he was taking home and on his way he had to cross a plank over .... over a pond. He looked down and .... there was .... his own reflection in the water and he thought there .... in the water was another dog ... with the piece of meat. He thought he'd have that piece of meat to. ...... So he snatched at the dog .... but as he opened his mouth .... the piece of meat fell into the pond and was never seen again.

Case 20

A girl with a normal developmental history, from a bilingual Italian/English family, was admitted at the age of 11;6 years in an unconscious state, having been knocked down by a car on her way to school. She was unresponsive and her pupils were small. A CT scan performed as an emergency showed multiple contusions in the left anterior and the right posterior parts of the internal capsule, with possible blood in the right lateral ventricle. She also had a displaced fracture of the right tibia. She was admitted to the intensive care unit, ventilated and given intravenous mannitol. The EEG was not abnormal. Brain-stem and visual evoked responses showed increased latency. She was ventilated for 13 days, did not respond to commands and had marked dystonic movements, more on the left than on the right. She remained unchanged for 5 weeks when she suddenly started responding to commands and became less restless. She was mobile, could understand simple requests, had single word speech, and was eating and drinking well; she regained continence of urine and faeces within 1 week. She was discharged with a mild, right upper motor neurone, seventh nerve palsy, a tremor of the left hand which was worse on movement, a slightly broad-based gait and a moderate mixed dysphasia.

She returned to her previous mainstream secondary school but had considerable problems in language, learning and emotional stability. Within the large, mixed ability classes, in which it was difficult to give specific teaching help, she made very poor progress and became depressed. It was difficult for the family to attend local speech therapy appointments, even in the school holidays, and she therefore received little specific help. She continued to have a significant word-finding problem as well as a dysphonia, due to bilateral vocal fold weakness. Two years post-trauma, a statement of educational needs was made by which she received extra teaching help of 0.2 whole time equivalent (w.t.e.). She also received some out-patient treatment from the department of child and adolescent psychiatry.

Her responses on the Grading Naming Test (McKenna and Warrington, 1983) showed some of the naming difficulties she had (Table 9.3).

Table 9.3 Responses of Case 20 on the Graded Naming Test

Post-trauma (months)	Item	Response	Error type
3	Camel	Giraffe	Semantic paraphasia
	Goat	Giraffe	Perseveration
	Waterfall	Waterchute	Semantic paraphasia
9	Cup	Glass	Semantic paraphasia
29	Kangaroo	Giraffe	Semantic paraphasia

Her progress with story telling showed that she gradually became more fluent and was able to use longer sentences, shown with examples of the same Dog Story, the first one at 6 months post-onset:

> There was a dog walking with a piece of meat in his mouth. . . . . . . He saw another dog . . . . . with another piece of meat in his mouth. The meat fell out of his mouth.

Then again at 18 months post-onset:

> The dog was walking home with a piece of meat in his mouth . . . . and he crossed a plank . . . . and then saw a river and then saw his own reflection in the water and he thought it was another dog with another piece of meat in his mouth. . . . . and. . . and so er. . . . he. . he dropped the meat and it fell in the river and he never saw it again.

The following language sample revealed some of her feelings about her school placement and lack of friends. She complained of headaches and tiredness (common features of depression) and her

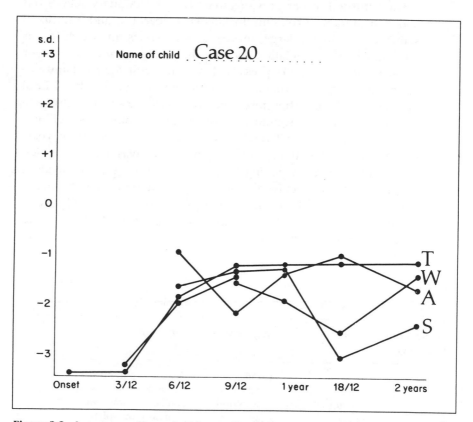

Figure 9.2 Language profile graph of Case 20. T = TROG; A = auditory association; S = sentence repetition; W = word finding

description of her comprehension difficulties was consistent with her test results. The difficulties she had with her written language included spelling and punctuation errors as well as some sentence formulation difficulties. This piece was written 1 year post-trauma.

> teachers sort of miss me in class, I have tried to ask to play but all of a sudden they give lies meant to hurt me. When I stay with Friend I (fel) stay happier to them and they think twice. When I'm in class and the teacher goes to Fast For me and I get mygrians and because of that I move about a lot and do the work wrong somet(h)imes. Work sheets I have to read over again and again until I get aroond to now what its (an) about. everyBody had a Friend to(e) go home with play with and do over things with. if it carrys on like this I with just (t go hom) leave. (Self-corrections in brackets, spelling and punctuation as original.)

Figure 9.2 shows the progress of Case 20 over 2 years.

The progress made by these two girls over the first 2 years after their head injuries was documented using the Test for Reception of Grammar (TROG; Bishop, 1983), and other measures of word finding, association naming and sentence repetition (Figures 9.1 and 9.2). It is clear that Case 19 made significantly better progress overall than Case 20. All the scores for Case 19 were within the normal range by the end of the first year. Case 20 continued to have z-scores in the range -1 to -2, and below, at 2 years post-trauma, which directly reflected the moderate to severe nature of her aphasia. In both cases the most consistent period of progress was during the first 6 months postinjury, after which progress gradually tailed off.

Not all children who suffer severe traumatic head injury will have severe residual aphasia or other communication difficulties. However, a complex range of speech and language problems is a common sequela to severe brain injury. Only comprehensive assessment carried out over time will reveal the nature of these problems and allow appropriate management to be planned.

Unilateral Cerebral Lesions

There are two major causes of acquired childhood aphasia in this group: vascular disease including cerebrovascular accident (CVA) and arterio-venous malformation (AVM), and cerebral infection causing cerebral abscess. It is difficult to separate completely those children with diffuse from those with focal cerebral lesions in clinical practice. Whilst it is clear that complex head injury is likely to have more diffuse effects there may be areas of additional focal damage. Equally, for the child who has a stroke or a cerebral abscess, the effect of which is essentially focal, other more diffuse damage may accompany this.

As with head injury, few studies have considered these aetiological groups exclusively. When considering acquired language problems in childhood, it is usual to include only those children whose cerebral lesions were obviously acquired after spoken language had become established. Children with congenital lesions may be included in the group described as cerebral palsied or occasionally those with developmental language disorders (see Case 10 in Chapter 3). This does of course leave a grey area, roughly between 6 and 18 months of age, when it is problematic to decide whether a child should be considered to have an acquired problem or not. The other important influence in the management of ACA is that acquired aphasia from unilateral cerebral lesions is much more common in adults. Thus, an adult-based model has dominated discussion in this area since Broca first described what is now called 'Broca's aphasia, in 1863. A number of researchers have tried to use adult-based classificatory systems to describe ACA. A recent study (Lees, 1989) of 34 children with ACA arising from a wide range of aetiologies suggests that the most commonly used system in adult aphasia (Goodglass and Kaplan, 1972) fails to classify most children with ACA. It is interesting that its application in adult aphasia has also been questioned (Marshall, 1986).

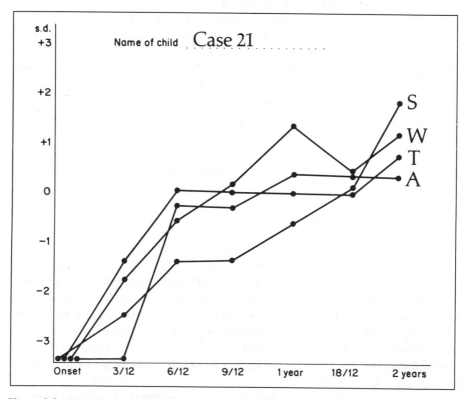

Figure 9.3 Language profile graph of Case 21. T = TROG; A = auditory association; S = sentence repetition; W = word finding

The effect of an acquired vascular lesion on a child's language does appear to vary considerably from child to child. Factors such as site of lesion, age at which the lesion is acquired and the initial severity of the disorder have been suggested as the major variables related to prognosis. The way in which these variables interact is not understood but, as with developmental language disorder, it is obviously far from simple. Cases 21 and 22 are the cases of two girls who had lesions of the left hemisphere at different ages, all of which resulted in a severe acute aphasia, but who demonstrate this variability of recovery quite well. The first did very well to recover from a complete aphasia at the age of 13 years. At the age of 17 she had a mild high level language problem in speed and volume of processing and recall, and a risk of epilepsy. The recovery of the second child's language was slower. She had greater residual language problems and a severe right hemiplegia. Whilst they do not represent all the possible outcomes for this group they do demonstrate some of the variability which is encountered. Profiles of the recovery of these children are given in Figures 9.3 and 9.4.

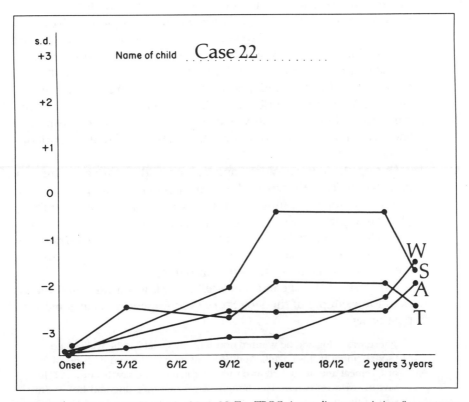

Figure 9.4 Language profile graph of Case 22. T = TROG; A = auditory association; S = sentence repetition; W = word finding

Case 21

This case is of a girl with a normal developmental history who presented with an acute aphasia at 13 years of age. CT scan and angiography revealed a large posterior temporoparietal haemorrhage from an AVM. There was a right hemianopia and very mild incoordination on the right. Initially she had a severe deficit in both receptive and expressive language, could comprehend only single nouns and produced both semantic and phonemic paraphasias. Pure-tone audiometry confirmed normal hearing. On discharge from hospital, she continued to receive speech therapy from her local service once weekly for at least a year. Eleven months post-onset she was readmitted with a small episode of language disturbance following a severe and prolonged headache, and some right-sided signs. There was a deterioration in her auditory–verbal processing and an increase in paraphasias. This appeared to resolve within 1 week. Two years after the intial event, another short episode of the same kind occurred; she was treated with carbamazepine and had stereotactic radiotherapy to a residual piece of the original AVM deep in the left temporal lobe. Her full scale WISC IQ taken 1 month after the first episode was 76, and 1 year later it had improved to 96. She had a statement of educational needs which made provision for a personal tutor and integration to mainstream comprehensive school. By the age of 17 years she had passed three GSCE examinations and was studying for three more. She continued to experience high level difficulties in the verbal comprehension of complex instructions in a noisy environment and occasional word-finding problems. She remained on anticonvulsants.

During the course of her aphasia she did produce a range of paraphasias. These were predominantly phonemic and an increase always accompanied subsequent episodes. Some examples of these phonemic paraphasias include (2 months post-onset): 'scarecrow' was called 'scarescrow', 'handcuffs' were 'handcrups', 'sporran' was called 'skoran'. Similar errors occurred over the next 2 years but there were never more than this in one session.

Expressive language in a story-telling task was always non-fluent as in the example of the Dog Story (see Appendix II) at 3 months post-onset:

> There was a dog and he wented down to the canal and he walked a p . . . (six attempts at this) plank. And he went down . . he and with his piece of . . . . meat and he looked into the . . . . canal and he saw his new . . . . he saw his own reflection. He thought it was another dog and he . . . did sort of throw . . . he dived in dived in and he never s . . . and he never saw his meat again.

Case 22

This is the case of a girl with a normal developmental history who presented with an acute aphasia at 8;3 years, and with a right hemiplegia. CT scan and angiography revealed severe arterial disease involving the left terminal internal carotid, left proximal middle cerebral artery and distal middle cerebral artery, with a large infarct. Pure-tone audiometry confirmed a mild conductive hearing loss of less than 30 dB which was of long standing. She had a severe receptive and expressive aphasia such that she did not even respond to single words, and she was essentially anomic. There was some improvement in all areas but 3 years post-onset she remained severely language disabled. She continued to receive speech therapy on a weekly basis from her local service for 2 years post-onset; the right hemiplegia persisted. Six months post-onset her WISC IQ was recorded as 86 on the Performance Scale and 52 on the Verbal Scale. No alternative provision for her educational needs was made by the local authority and she continued in a mainstream comprehensive school where she made very poor progress. Her right hemiplegia also persisted unchanged.

She produced very little language, and was particularly reluctant to name items to confrontation. Therefore, few naming errors were recorded and those few given here suggest a general naming impairment (at 3 months post-onset): 'basket' was called 'purse' as was 'case', 'saw' was called 'knife'.

Very little spontaneous expressive language ever occurred but some short phrases were produced in a story-telling situation. This example of the Farmer Story was recorded 9 months post-onset:

> The farmer and the donkey go in barn. He pushed him . . . . . He pulled him . . . . no go. Tell the cat scratch dog. Cat scratch him. Dog bark. He went in barn.

The paraphasic naming errors reported in these cases are consistent with other recent reports in the literature. Van Hout, Everard and Lyon (1985) documented a series of cases demonstrating a wide range of paraphasias, both as temporary initial features of the aphasia and as more persistent long-term problems. In the 11 children aged 4 to 10 years they discussed, semantic or phonemic paraphasias always occurred. The tendency to perseverate these naming errors was also reported as quite a frequent occurrence. They postulated that the lack of previous reports of paraphasia in cases of ACA of this kind (essentially the view before 1978) may have been due to the fact that language investigations were not always carried out as soon as was reasonably possible. Where the paraphasic period was short (perhaps only a few days), they would therefore have been missed. Clinical experiences of seeing children from acute onset to long-term follow-up supports the view that detailed assessment at all stages of recovery is important for a full understanding of ACA. Lees (1989) reported that 79% of the children in her study produced paraphasic errors at some time during the recovery period. These data further supported Van Hout, Everard and Lyon (1985) that a paraphasic period of longer than 6 months was a poor prognostic sign.

When determining the need for intervention directed at the child's naming difficulties an analysis of the types of cues the child generates or finds helpful when supplied by others is an important consideration. Children and adults without language problems use self-generated and other cues to aid naming when necessary. It is possible to help the aphasic child regain an understanding of cueing. By observing which cues the child finds most helpful, a programme to reinforce these in a range of naming and other tasks can be prepared. Initially tasks will involve naming in a structured but non-pressurised situation. Gradually the structure can be altered to include recall of names in other situations, including group tasks and more informal tasks or timed tasks. The child may be encouraged to keep a note book, where possible, to record situations in which naming proved difficult for later discussions with the therapist. These can then be re-enacted in a role play and the child can work through the range of strategies which would help naming if a similar situation were to recur.

Cerebral Abscess

The most likely cause of cerebral infection which can result in language impairment is an intracranial abscess in the left hemisphere resulting in a focal lesion. Meningitis and encephalitis (see Appendix I) can underlie acquired language disorders in children, but the results are often rather different. First, because coma is a common sequela to the more severe forms of cerebral infection, the result may be equally severe affecting motor and cognitive function as well as language. One of the reported sequelae of some types of meningitis is a high frequency deafness. All children who present with acquired aphasia should have a hearing test to establish audiological status. The competence of the auditory mechanism for effective language rehabilitation is just as important for children with developmental or acquired conditions.

In early studies of ACA (Guttman, 1942; Collignon, Hecaen and Angelergues, 1968) children with aphasia after cerebral abscess, particularly of the left temporal lobe, were common. This abscess usually arises as a complication of severe otitis media (see Appendix I) and mastoiditis (inflammation/infection of the mastoid bone), and affects the middle to posterior portion of the temporal lobe. Abscesses are less common with the use of antibiotics to treat otitis media. Another area which is vulnerable to infection is the frontal lobes. Here an abscess may follow frontal sinusitis

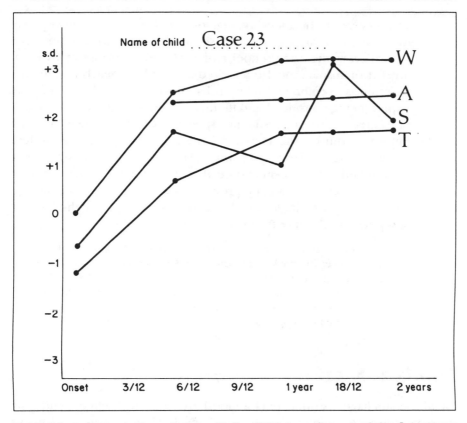

Figure 9.5 Language profile graph of Case 23. T = TROG; A = auditory association; S = sentence repetition; W = word finding

and, where the dominant hemisphere is involved, aphasia can be part of the presenting symptoms. Treatment usually involves surgical draining of the abscess and antibiotics for the infection. Cerebral abscess has not been a frequent contributor to cases of aphasia we have treated. Case 23 is one example of an older teenager who made a good recovery from a mild aphasia (Figure 9.5).

Case 23

A boy with a normal developmental history presented with acute aphasia at 15 years of age. CT scan revealed frontal cortical damage following the anterior medial frontal lobe and laterally round to the centro-sylvian region (i.e. involving the parietal lobe) secondary to a subdural abscess which was drained. There was no infarct and the damage would appear to have been purely cortical. Pure-tone audiometry confirmed normal hearing. The IQ before illness (at age 11 years) had been tested for educational placement and was said to be above average on the WISC; this would appear to have been preserved because he returned to continue his education at the same school and achieved 11 passes at GCE 'O' level at the usual time. He received a period of speech therapy for 3 months beginning 6 months post-onset. when he was experiencing considerable difficulty in initiating some sounds and presented with a dysfluent speech pattern. However, this improved during the course of therapy and was more or less unnoticeable 1 year post-onset. He never had a significant comprehension problem and he also did not produce paraphasias. Once the initial dysfluency problem was overcome, his language soon returned to its former level as this example of the Farmer Story recorded 6 months post-onset shows:

> There once was a farmer, who owned a stubborn donkey. The farmer wanted to get the donkey into the barn. First he pushed him, then he pulled him, but the donkey would not move. So he asked the dog to bark so he could frighten the donkey into the barn, but the lazy dog refused. So he asked the cat to make it bark. The cat was cooperative and scratched the dog. The dog barked and the barking frightened the donkey so that he jumped into the barn.

Landau–Kleffner Syndrome

Of all the language disorders of childhood, the Landau–Kleffner syndrome must rank among the most puzzling. It is probably the rarest, and many paediatric speech therapists will never have seen a case. First described by Landau and Kleffner in 1957, it is also called acquired aphasia with convulsive disorder and acquired receptive aphasia. These names refer to the co-occurring neurological disorder and the predominantly receptive language difficulty.

In this type of aphasia, language regresses after a period of normal language development. Typically, this is usually receptive language initially followed by expressive language. There is often an accompanying seizure disorder, or the condition may be preceded by seizures. However, in about one-third of reported cases there are never any seizures. In the original paper by Landau and Kleffner (1957) six children aged 5–9 years were described. Whilst their description of the presenting language problem is not detailed, a wide range of associated epileptic phenomena are described, both focal and generalised. In two of the children, there was a family history of epilepsy and, in two others, a recent previous history of mild head injury. Three of the children had a history of more than one period of aphasia and their condition appeared to have had a fluctuating course. The body of literature on acquired childhood aphasia from Landau–Kleffner syndrome contains both small group studies, single case descriptions and several retrospective analyses of previously reported cases, but our knowledge of the pathological mechanism underlying the disorder, and our ability to predict prognosis or treat the condition medically remain uncertain. Dugas et al. (1976) reported a case in which the administration of anti-epileptic treatment was followed by considerable improvement in the language disorder, but cases like this do not form the majority of those published. It was the clinical variability that led Deonna et al. (1977) to suggest that the Landau–Kleffner syndrome was a heterogeneous syndrome with at least three courses:

1. Rapid onset of language disorder followed by rapid recovery, with a good prognosis.
2. Repeated seizures and gradual worsening of the aphasia, with subsequent aphasic periods, and variable recovery.
3. Progressively deteriorating language, no seizures and variable recovery.

The variable clinical picture has led to some debate about the core features of the condition, the typical course and the most effective management. It has been suggested that such a wide range of possibilities is hardly likely to represent one syndrome. Moreover, because the condition has rarely been comprehensively described from the language point of view, an equally wide range of reports about the possible presenting language symptoms exists. It is considered to be a predominantly receptive disorder, and some describe this as a verbal auditory agnosia (Cooper and Ferry, 1978). Others concentrate on the expressive language features and report word-finding difficulties and paraphasic errors (Dugas et al., 1976; Van der Sandt-Koenderman et al., 1984). Case 24 describes a fairly typical course which would fall into the third group, as defined by Deonna et al. (1977).

Case 24

A girl presented at the age of 6;9 years with a history of a slow deterioration in language skills that had begun 9 months previously. Prior to this she had been developing normally and had attended a mainstream infant school. There was no family history of speech and language problems. She had no history of epilepsy. Initially, the problem had been thought of as a fluctuating hearing loss, but all audiological investigations were normal. By the time she was referred for this assessment she was only comprehending simple phrases in situational context. Her expressive language was also reduced to simple stereotyped phrases. The school reported that her behaviour was difficult to manage. Neurological examination was normal throughout, as was a CT scan. EEG revealed a focus of abnormal activity in the left temporal lobe, but there were

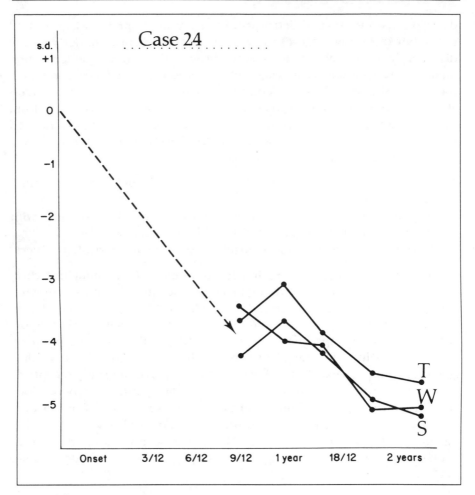

Figure 9.6 Language profile graph of Case 24. T = TROG; S = sentence repetition; W = word finding; ---- marks presumed course of deterioration

no overt fits. She did complain of not sleeping well and a pain in her left ear but nothing could be found to explain this. Her IQ on the WISC(R) was 71 on the Full Scale, 91 on Performance Scale and 55 on Verbal Scale. She passed two blocks on the TROG, comprehending single nouns and single verbs only. She produced a number of naming errors on the WFVT, which were often irrelevant stereotypes or requests for her mother to respond on her behalf. The changes in these tests scores over the following years are shown in Figure 9.6. A trial of carbamazepine was begun to see if verbal comprehension would improve, but it was unchanged 6 weeks later. A trial of steroids was introduced instead and discontinued 6 weeks later when verbal comprehension still remained unchanged, although behaviour further deteriorated. After this all anticonvulsants were withdrawn without further effect.

It was clear from observations of her at school and home that she was comprehending very little. Her deteriorating behaviour was directly related to her failure to comprehend. She was reluctant to be parted from her mother and relied heavily on her for 'translation' of what was happening or being said. She would turn her mother's face towards her when she wanted such an explanation and also used the same technique if she was trying to tell her mother something. This behaviour is fairly common in young language-disordered children with severe comprehension problems. A statement of educational need was drawn up and she was placed in a language unit at the age of 7;4 years. Her verbal comprehension remained unchanged over the course of the following 6 months. A system of language teaching through reading based on the Colour Pattern Scheme (Lea, 1970) was used to work on visual comprehension of language structure. Listening and attention work were also encouraged as was basic sentence construction work. With no change in her verbal comprehension, it is clear that she is likely to require long-term placement in a school for children with speech and language disorders.

Variations on this theme are almost as many as there are children presenting with the condition, which does suggest that the effects of cerebral dysfunction during language development cannot be confined to simplistic views about locality of lesion (especially as these children rarely show significant lesions on CT scan), the age of the child at onset, the initial severity of the language problem or the co-occurrance of other neurological symptoms. Once again a complex interrelationship between these factors is suggested by the clinical evidence. Dulac, Billard and Arthuis (1983) have suggested that paroxysmal discharges act in some way to block access to the language areas of the cortex. This hypothesis bears some relation to the phenomenon of aphasic arrest, described by Penfield and Rasmussen (1950) in their studies of adults undergoing electrical stimulation of the cortex during neurosurgery for intractable epilepsy. Bishop (1985) reviewed 45 cases from the literature in order to discuss the variable age of onset in relation to outcome. She agreed with the widely held clinical view that the older the child at onset the better the prognosis. This is the opposite to the position in children with aphasia from unilateral cerebral lesions, in whom prognosis for recovery is poorer with increasing age.

Several years of seeing children with this syndrome in clinical practice has resulted in data from a small but highly variable group of children (some of this group are reported in Lees, 1989). They have ranged in age from 2 to 12 years at onset. Some have presented acutely, and in others there has been a period of language deterioration lasting several weeks to several months. Those with the longer period of deterioration seem to have a poorer prognosis. Complete verbal auditory agnosia has been seen in a number of cases. However, this is not always the major symptom. The receptive language component may fluctuate, whereas in others verbal language is absent or considerably reduced. Older children may present with a rather pedantic conversational style with inappropriate prosody. Data from Lees (1989) suggest that children who do not make progress to within −2 standard deviations in verbal comprehension within 6 months of onset are in the poor outcome group. Most of these children will require special educational provision within a specialised teaching environment in which visual methods of teaching language (signing and reading) are backed up with a lot of work on useful communication for everyday life.

Conclusions about Acquired Childhood Aphasia

The aim of these case descriptions was to outline the features of language impairment in ACA, the evolution of such language problems and the way in which speech therapists, who may not be so familiar with the disorder, might assess them. Thus, each description contained a graph to demonstrate the change in test scores during the course of recovery and clinical descriptions of the range of problems the children presented with. These clinical descriptions included details of the neurological, psychological, audiological and educational status of the children to give as full a picture as possible of aphasic language in childhood. This combination of objective measure and clinical description is a reflection of the way in which speech therapists set out to differentiate language problems in clinical practice. We have aimed to formalise this throughout the book in order to demonstrate the value of this practical method.

The main conclusions which should be drawn here about ACA concern three main points: the features of the disorders, the question of recovery and the application to speech therapy.

The features of acquired childhood aphasia

The traditional view of ACA, that ACA from trauma was predominantly an expressive problem and ACA from Landau–Kleffner syndrome predominantly a receptive one, has not been borne out by recent studies. Children in both groups present with a wide range of deviant language behaviours. In the Lees (1989) study, there was a high incidence of acute auditory comprehension problems (78%) and word-finding difficulties (58%), revealing both receptive and expressive problems in both groups. The majority of the children (79%) produced paraphasias at some stage during their recovery. A substantial minority also made perseverated errors or had difficulties with the form and fluency of expressive language. These must all be recognised as possible features of ACA since a substantial number of other studies, many of them of smaller numbers, have also reported them (Van Dongen, Loonen and Van Dongen, 1985; Van Hout, Evrard and Lyon, 1985). Pure acute expressive aphasia appears to be rare, and high level receptive problems often persist.

Further, Lees (1989) stated that classification of the children's language problems using the system advocated by Goodglass and Kaplan (1972) to differentiate aphasic syndromes suggested that the features of ACA rarely fall into the same subtypes, either in the acute or the long-term stages. Half the children could not be categorised using this terminology. The classification of children with ACA awaits the development of a better system for the classification of all types of language disorders in childhood.

The question of recovery from acquired childhood aphasia

The traditional view of a good recovery from traumatic aphasia in childhood being the usual course of the disorder has not been borne out by recent studies (Cooper and Flowers, 1987; Jordan, Ozanne and Murdoch, 1988; Lees, 1989). Although children showed improvement during the course of all these studies, and some even regained the normal range on some of the tests used, few could be said to have had no residual problems. Even when these were mild, high level problems, they could not be presumed to be insignificant. According to Lees (1989), the period of fastest recovery was during the first 3 months after onset. Children who recovered to pass the level of −2 standard deviations within 6 months of onset continued to do well. Those that did not make this amount of progress in that time had a poorer prognosis. The persistence of deviant language features, particularly paraphasias and perseveration after 1 year, was also a poor prognostic sign.

The language tests detailed earlier have proved useful as a basic battery for the assessment of ACA. However, they are not altogether able to define residual high level difficulties, which may only be apparent from the reports of the child, parents or teachers. The practice of regular detailed assessment over time can help to establish the changing profile of language disorder which may help when planning appropriate management, including medical, educational and therapeutic intervention.

The children discussed here do not represent a fully comprehensive account of the language problems seen during recovery from ACA. It is clear from the range reported in the literature, that even when a fairly sizeable group is described (Lees, 1989) or a number of papers summarised (Bishop, 1985), the variability in ACA is considerable. Future work in this field may include a larger study to look at the question of relationship between specific language deficits and aetiology of aphasia. Armed with information about the natural history of ACA, we are in a better position to decide when a period of intervention might be planned. A suitable assessment battery allows us to establish which specific deficits require attention. Other future work may also be a series of studies, probably using a single case design, into the effects of particular types of treatment for children with residual language problems. However, such work probably awaits reporting in a more detailed study devoted to ACA.

ACA is not a common cause of language difficulty in childhood, and has not therefore attracted a great deal of attention from those interested in language-disordered children. Because of the smaller numbers of children involved, and the previously common belief that most made a good recovery, ACA has been seen as a fringe issue in understanding language impairment in childhood. However, the advantages of studying this group are that the criteria for entry are clear (as opposed to the definition by exclusion that has commonly been used for developmental language disorder), the group is small and therefore manageable and the condition presents a natural experiment in that a reasonable amount of recovery is the normal course of the disorder. Comprehensive assessment and follow-up of children with ACA over 2 years (Lees, 1989) has established the value of appropriate longitudinal assessment to document the course of the disorder. The range of features which children present with, the practice of diagnosing complex language problems in association with other professionals, the selection of children for treatment and the discussion of prognosis with and without treatment were some of the other issues this study addressed.

We still have a great deal to learn about ACA and related conditions in which skills are lost in childhood. In many of these syndromes the mechanisms underlying the deterioration are very poorly understood. Determining prognosis is often difficult and in many cases the outlook is poor. Managing ACA is the proper concern of a multidisciplinary team including at least a speech therapist, paediatrician/paediatric neurologist (as appropriate), educational psychologist, teacher and the child's family. These can be confusing and distressing disorders, both acutely and in the long term. Further research into cause(s) and treatment are required. Meanwhile it is important to emphasise that ACA, whilst less common than developmental language disorder, is not 'a fringe issue'. For the children and their families, appropriate action is important during the various stages of recovery. We cannot afford just to wait and see if the child gets better. Rehabilitation services for head-injured children and structured language programmes for those with receptive aphasia need to be planned.

Appendix I
Some Syndromes and Conditions associated with Language Impairment

Summary

A number of syndromes which are associated with speech and language impairment are outlined. Information concerning the aetiology, course and management of these disorders is briefly summarised and relevant research findings are discussed.

Asperger's Syndrome

This was first described by Asperger in 1944. He described a condition he called 'autistic psychopathy' in children and it is now generally recognised to be one subtype of the pervasive developmental disorders, of which infantile autism is another. Broadly speaking, the clinical features of the disorder are social isolation, abnormal interaction with peers, impaired non-verbal and verbal communication and early developmental delays (Wing, 1981). However, some researchers have found it more difficult to distinguish the condition from autism and consider Asperger's syndrome to be a mild variant of that disorder. Others have concentrated on the presenting features of language difficulty and have tended to refer to a semantic–pragmatic language disorder. The notion that this condition may overlap or form part of a spectrum is discussed by Bishop (1989). Most clinicians now use the term 'Asperger's syndrome' to refer to children who have a major social impairment, in association with difficulties in language and cognitive development, but who do not fit the usual category of autism and whose problems appear to be at a higher (more subtle) level.

Cerebral Palsy

This is a disorder of movement and posture due to a defect or lesion of the immature brain (Bax, 1964). The lesion and the disorder are non-progressive. It may arise prenatally, at the time of birth, or in the neonatal period. The major result is an impairment of coordination so that the child is unable to perform the usual range of movements or maintain posture. There may be associated problems in the motor movements of speech. The actual manifestations of the disorder will depend on which parts of the motor system are affected. In its severest form, it affects all four limbs (quadriplegia). It may be more severe in the lower limbs (diplegia) or on one side (hemiplegia – see below). Other deficits arising from central nervous system dysfunction may occur, including visual and hearing problems, perceptual or sensory disturbances, problems with cognitive development and epilepsy.

Cleft Palate

Clefts of the lip and palate are among the most commonly occurring congenital abnormalities. Cleft lip without cleft palate occurs in approximately 1:1000 live births. It is the result of a failure in the fusion of the lip at 35 days of uterine life. The occurrence of cleft lip and palate together is the most common oral clefting syndrome and accounts for approximately 50% of all cases. It is twice as frequent in males as in females. A cleft may be unilateral or bilateral, and in unilateral cases the left side is twice as likely to be affected as the right. Repeated otitis media is a common consequence of cleft palate. This is due to palatal incompetence and a failure of the levator palatine muscle to effectively control the opening of the pharyngeal end of the eustachian tube which aerates the middle ear.

Cocktail Party Syndrome

This is a particular kind of language impairment which has been asssociated with hydrocephalus in children. It is said to be a language development profile in which, in children of low intelligence, language skills appear disproportionately good. Long and complex sentences are used which include advanced vocabulary items. However, the children usually have poor comprehension and much of their language is found to be irrelevant or lacking in content. The name 'cocktail party' is related to the empty nature of the conversation, said to be reminiscent of the kind of conversation conducted over cocktails. Not all children with hydrocephalus are found to demonstrate this language profile.

Down's Syndrome

First described by Down (1866), he called the condition mongolism or mongoloid idiocy. The term 'Down's syndrome' is now preferred. It is a chromosome disorder affecting approximately one in 800 live births. It is a common cause of severe mental handicap accounting for about one-third of that population. About 20% of Down's syndrome infants die from associated anomalies in the first 2 years of life. Three different subtypes of the chromosome abnormality have been identified. In the standard condition, called trisomy 21, chromosome no. 21 has three copies instead of two in all cells in the body. This subtype accounts for about 95% of all cases of Down's syndrome. About 4% are termed 'translocations'. Here extra chromosome material is also found in all cells, but the mechanism by which it arises is different. The remaining 1% are termed 'mosaicism'. In these cases only certain types of cells contain the extra chromosomes and the rest have the usual number. It is important to emphasise the considerable variability of development which occurs in Down's syndrome. However, it is not yet known how these various chromosomal subtypes account for these variations in development. At birth, hypotonia (floppiness) is common. Most Down's syndrome children walk late, at around 24 months. Speech and language development is also usually delayed to between 2;6 to 4 years for first words. A range of other problems may also occur, including congenital heart defects and severe learning difficulties.

Encephalitis

This is a viral infection affecting the brain and the spinal cord. The number of viruses which are known to attack the central nervous system is large. They may be transmitted in a number of ways – by human contact, by insects or other animal contacts. Encephalitis can occur at any age but is most common in childhood, adolescence and young adulthood. Symptoms vary, but the most characteristic onset is a mild febrile illness; headache and drowsiness are common. In more severe cases, this develops to confusion and eventually coma. In younger children convulsions commonly co-occur, and there may also be a range of motor and sensory changes which can be mild or include complete paralysis. Recovery is also variable with some forms of encephalitis having a higher mortality or morbidity rate than others.

Epilepsies of Childhood

It is said that 3–7% of all children will have one or more epileptic seizure before the age of 5 years (Acardi and Chevrie, 1986). Epileptic seizures are evidence of cerebral dysfunction, and usually arise from structural or physiological abnormalities of the brain. Clinically, they give rise to changes in consciousness, behaviour, and disturbances of motor and autonomic activity. The international classification of epilepsy, which was most recently revised in 1981, divides epileptic seizures into three groups: generalised seizures, partial seizures and unclassified seizures. However, there is no accepted system of classifying epilepsy (as opposed to classifying the types of seizures observed). Five main groups of epilepsies have been suggested: generalised convulsions (called primary if related to physiological abnormalities and secondary when associated with cerebral lesions), partial epilepsies (in which partial and/or unilateral seizures may occur which may be motor, sensory, autonomic or psychic phenomena), absence epilepsies, myoclonic epilepsies (in which a certain type of movements, called myoclonic, is seen) and epileptic syndromes, including the Lennox–Gestaut syndrome, West's syndrome (also called infantile spasms) and the Landau–Kleffner syndrome. Febrile convulsions are seizures which occur between 5 months and 5 years of age with fever (where the fever is not related to cerebral infection or other cerebral disorder). They are generally considered to be benign with a recurrence risk of 30–40%. The risk of the child going on to develop further epilepsy is put at about 5%. Epilepsy is more commonly seen in children with learning difficulties. Corbett (1985) gives figures of 6% (in children with an IQ of 50–70) to nearly 50% (in those with an IQ below 20) prevalence. For children with specific language difficulties, Robinson (1987) reports 21% with definite seizures and a further 11% who had a questionable history of seizures. He stated a belief that there is a particular association between epilepsy and language disorder, but this is not understood.

Fragile X Syndrome

This syndrome, associated with an abnormality of the end of the long arm of the X chromosome called a fragile site, is one of a large group of syndromes in the X-linked recessive mental handicap group (Lubs, 1983). The affected males have a characteristic appearance, including large ears, a prominent forehead and large testes. At birth the head is often very large (up to the 97th centile), but it is within the average range in older children and adults. Some of those affected have large hands. The characteristic language disorder which has been described is said to be largely expressive such that speech is jocular and repetitive in style. Stuttering may also occur. The syndrome has also been described in about 7% of mildly mentally handicapped females.

Hemiplegia

Sometimes divided into congenital hemiplegia (present from birth) and infantile hemiplegia (acquired during early childhood), the most common cause is a cerebrovascular lesion. This may be associated with prematurity, but more usually with a cerebral abnormality like an angioma or other lesion, the cause of which may be unknown. In acquired cases hemiplegia may be associated with an encephalitis or meningitis (see other references in this section) or with cerebral tumour or convulsions. Hemiplegia is essentially a motor disorder affecting one side of the body, which arises from an upper motor neurone lesion. Although both gross and fine motor skills would seem to be the obvious considerations for the child's development, other problems may co-occur. Where there is epilepsy, there is a greater risk of learning difficulties. Speech and language development may also be delayed or disordered. It has generally been thought that the latter is more likely when the hemiplegia is on the right side, but cases of left hemiplegia with language disorder should not be overlooked, particularly where epilepsy may be a contributing factor.

Hydrocephalus

This refers to an excess of cerebrospinal fluid (CSF; that fluid surrounding the brain and spinal cord) resulting in a dilatation of the ventricular system. In children it may be acquired or congenital. Congenital hydrocephalus is usually due to a congenital malformation interfering with circulation of the CSF. It is commonly associated with spina bifida and sometimes with severe birth trauma. Acquired hydrocephalus may be due to a tumour in the third or fourth ventricle which interrupts the flow of CSF. The most noticeable symptoms of hydrocephalus is the size of the head. This is usually noticed in the first few months of life in congenital cases. Diagnosis relies on consistent and accurate measurements of head circumference. Other signs include the widening of the cranial sutures and the enlargement of the anterior fontanelle. In acquired cases the symptoms are more variable. Commonly they include headache, vomiting and sometimes impaired consciousness. Other mild neurological signs may include weakness and incoordination of the limbs. Congenital hydrocephalus is commonly associated with learning difficulties and epilepsy. In acquired cases the prognosis will depend on the original cause. In both types treatment is surgical and usually involves fitting a valve which then regulates the pressure of the CSF and sometimes the removal of the obstruction. However, sometimes hydrocephalus 'arrests', i.e. the head circumference stops growing. Hydrocephalus in children has previously been thought to be related to a particular communication style termed 'cocktail party syndrome'.

Incontinentia Pigmenti

Also called the Bloch–Sulzbeger syndrome and the Bloch–Siemens syndrome, this is an inherited condition which affects the skin, the eyes, and the skeletal and central nervous systems. Genetic evidence suggests that it is caused by a sex-related dominant gene. Almost all cases are female and incomplete forms of the syndrome may be found in some female relatives. The changes in the skin are often present at birth and have usually developed in the first week of life. There may be pigmented areas and warty eruptions. There is frequently delayed eruption of dentition, with partial anodontia. Teeth which are present are usually cone- or peg-shaped. Both deciduous and permanent teeth are abnormal. Cerebral atrophy may be seen on CT scan (Avrahami et al., 1985) and is related to developmental delay which is found in up to 50% of cases. Seizure disorders may also begin in the neonatal period or in later childhood. Early onset of seizures is usually related to a poor prognosis.

Infantile Autism

This was first described by Kanner in 1943, who presented a series of eleven cases (eight boys and three girls) to represent the usual range of the syndrome. He commented on five particular aspects of the development of these children: (1) inability to relate to other people as an early developmental difficulty, (2) failure to develop normal communication skills, (3) a range of abnormal responses to things in the child's environment (objects and events) which appeared to be governed by an obsessive desire for sameness, (4) some good cognitive abilities particularly with rote learning, memory and form boards, and (5) normal physical development. The syndrome was further defined by Rutter (1978a) who emphasised the distinction between general mental handicap and autism. He recommended the adoption of four criteria for the diagnosis of autism in children under 5 years. These were: onset of the disorder was before 30 months of age; there was a specific impairment of social development not consistent with intellectual development; the particular pattern of disordered language development was also inconsistent with intellectual development; and there was an obsession for sameness which was demonstrated by stereotyped play, a resistance to change and preoccupations. The debate as to what is and what is not autism or any one of its associated syndromes continues and is likely to do so whilst the diagnosis remains a clinical one. It has been suggested that the pattern of language disorder consistent with autism is a semantic–pragmatic one. However, other authors, notably Rapin and Allen (1987) confirm that other language-disorder patterns can be seen in individuals with autism and that not all children who present with semantic–pragmatic language disorders are also autistic.

Klinefelter's Syndrome

This syndrome was first described by Klinefelter, Reifenstein and Albright in 1942. It is also called XXY syndrome, which indicates that it is an abnormality of the sex chromosomes. It is thought to be the most common cause of infertility among males, affecting approximately 1:500. Other features of the condition are a tendency to tall growth in childhood and obesity in adulthood, small penis and testes, and learning difficulties. Onset of speech is generally late and problems of expressive language, including both articulatory and naming difficulties, have been described.

Landau–Kleffner Syndrome

First described by Landau and Kleffner in 1957, this is also called acquired receptive aphasia or acquired aphasia with convulsive disorder. It is a rare and poorly understood cause of language disorder. About one-third of the children never have seizures and in those that do the control of epilepsy is rarely a major problem. The major feature of the disorder is a deterioration in receptive language skills which can be either acute or happen over a prolonged period. In some cases it is preceded by a viral infection, epilepsy or minor head trauma, but the mechanism of cerebral dysfunction underlying the disorder is unknown. Where loss of receptive language is total over a long period and little recovery takes place, then the long-term prognosis is poor. However, a more acute onset with a fluctuating course appears to be related to a better prognosis.

Meningitis

This is an infection, usually bacterial, of the meninges usually involving the subarachnoid space and the cerebrospinal fluid. There are three ways in which this infection occurs: from the extension of a pre-existing infection usually of the sinuses or mastoid, from infection through the blood stream or after fracture of the skull. The onset may be quite dramatic and the first symptom is usually headache accompanied by fever. Vomiting may occur in the early stages and convulsions are common in children. The child may become delirious and then drowsy followed by coma. The prognosis generally depends on the effectiveness of the antibiotics used against the infection. The mortality rate among children varies and depends largely on the infecting organism. Other serious sequelae can include deafness, cerebral palsy and mental handicap.

Moebius' Syndrome

The usual feature of this syndrome is a mask-like face due to bilateral sixth and seventh nerve palsy. A small mandible is a frequent feature. There may also be evidence of involvement of other cranial nerves in some cases (including third, fourth, fifth, ninth, tenth and twelfth). The tongue may be small and of limited mobility. Feeding difficulties and problems of aspiration often lead to failure to thrive in early infancy. About 15% of those affected also have learning difficulties which suggests that cerebral involvement extends beyond the cranial nerve nuclei.

Muscular Dystrophy

The muscular dystrophies are a group of disorders in which the common feature is a progressive degeneration of muscles. The most common variety is Duchenne muscular dystrophy which is an inherited sex-linked recessive condition. Usually appearing about middle childhood, it occurs almost exclusively in boys. There is a gradual onset of difficulty or clumsiness in walking, a tendency to fall and a difficulty in getting up unaided. On examination it is usual to find some muscle groups to be enlarged and others wasted. The enlarged muscles are commonly in the calves, the buttocks and the shoulders and occasionally the forearms; chest muscles are often wasted. There is a waddling gait. Most affected individuals die in their teens.

Neurofibromatosis

Also called von Recklinghausen's disease, this is an inherited autosomal dominant condition. However, the extent and severity will differ within the same family. There are pigmented patches on the skin and tumours of the peripheral nerves (neurofibroma) and the skin (cutaneous fibroma). Neurofibromas may also occur in the spinal nerve roots. The most common and most constant symptoms are the patches of brownish spots (café-au-lait) on the skin; these range in size from a small spot to large patches.

Noonan's Syndrome

First described by Noonan and Ehmke (1963), this is a congenital disorder of which the major features are a range of heart abnormalities, developmental delay and a characteristic facial appearance. Few reports fully document the associated difficulties or oral function, hearing, speech and language development (Hopkins-Acos and Bunker, 1979; Wilson and Dyson, 1982; both report one child each). Quite severe feeding difficulties are commonly encountered. Delayed speech and language development has been reported, but specific areas of difficulty encountered by this group have not yet been accounted for. Although learning difficulties have been reported, the range of intelligence documented is wide. A comprehensive study of the development of oral function, speech and language in this condition is presently in progress.*

---

* A profile of the speech, language and feeding development in children with Noonan's syndrome is being prepared by J. Lees and D. Cave at the Department of Clinical Genetics, St George's Hospital Medical School, London.

Otitis Media

Probably one of the most common medical problems seen in children, this is an inflammation of the middle ear. The middle ear is an air-filled chamber between the tympanic membrane and the oval window, and it contains the ossicles. Otitis media is the most common cause of conductive hearing loss in children. Inflammation of the middle ear is due to bacterial or viral infection. Dysfunction or obstruction of the eustachian tube (from the middle ear to the pharynx) means that the chamber fills with fluid and this accumulates. With fluid in the cavity, the transmission of sound energy via the ossicles to the inner ear is disrupted. The fluid may be reabsorbed and recur with a further infection at a later stage. This means that the conductive hearing problem will fluctuate. Recurrent otitis media refers to repeated infections. The non-purulent fluid in the middle-ear cavity is sometimes termed 'glue ear'. Pus in the cavity is called suppurative otitis media.

Pierre Robin's Syndrome

This congenital disoder is considered to be due to an abnormality of the growth of the mandibular area which occurs before 9 weeks of fetal life. The mandible fails to develop properly which, in turn, affects the location of the tongue. This appears to locate in a more posterior position and impair the closure of the posterior palatal shelves, which must grow over the tongue to meet in the midline. The resulting cleft of the soft palate is usually more U-shaped than V-shaped (as in the usual facial clefting syndromes). The main problem faced by newborns is airway obstruction which may require pulling the tongue forward or nursing the infant in a head-down position. Early failure to thrive in association with feeding difficulties is not uncommon. Further growth of the palatal shelves may well occur, and surgery is often carried out between 3 and 4 years of age to allow for this (it is usually earlier in the facial clefting syndromes).

Rett's Syndrome

First described by Rett (1966), this is a severe form of learning disorder in which the onset is between 1 and 2 years. Criteria for diagnosing the syndrome include: female sex (there are no known cases who are males), early regression of behaviour, social and cognitive development so that skills gained appear to be lost, signs of dementia, loss of hand skills and the development of hand-writing stereotypies, the appearance of an ataxic gait and the deceleration of head growth. The most common misdiagnosis is with infantile autism. Children with Rett's syndrome do have stereotypical movements of the hands and poor social interactions. The characteristic hand-writhing movements frequently include putting the fingers or hands in the mouth; objects may also be mouthed persistently. The usual course of the condition is that it follows a fairly normal first year of life, although motor milestones may be slightly delayed. Cognitive development is usually normal for the first 9 months, and then slows down before regressing in the second year. A change in oral motor function has been reported from hypotonicity to hypertonicity, said to be directly related to postural changes, with fasciculating tongue movements and tongue deviations (more to the left than to the right) (Budden, Meek and Henighan, 1990). These authors also assessed the communication development in 20 girls, aged 3–19 years, none of whom demonstrated a level above 20 months. The resulting clinical picture is a profound mental handicap.

Sturge–Weber Syndrome

This is a capillary–venous malformation affecting one hemisphere and occurs in association with a facial naevus (port wine stain). This is congenital in origin and consists of a large mass of enlarged and twisted vessels which are supplied by one or more of the large cerebral arteries and drained by the large cerebral veins. It most commonly occurs supplied by the middle cerebral artery and arises from a failure in the embryonic development of the cerebral circulation. In the severest cases, the naevus may be quite large and extend from the face down the neck and arm. Epilepsy is commonly associated with this syndrome and the child may have a range of learning difficulties.

Treacher Collins Syndrome

A congenital condition in which the major features appear to be related to the fetal growth of the middle part of the face such that the mandible, zygomatic bone, lower eyelids, auricles, external ear canal and soft palate are the main parts of the face to be affected. Other anomalies include narrow respiratory passages and heart defects. The narrow airway may mean that tracheotomy is necessary in neonates. Learning difficulties are not a common association (only reported in 5% of cases). The recognition and correct management of the hearing problem (hearing aids, surgery and teaching) are usually the most important factors in the development of these children.

Williams' Syndrome

This is a rare metabolic disorder, the associated features of which are cardiac anomalies (most usually a narrowing of the aorta) and particular facial appearance described as 'elfin' and learning difficulties (as described by Williams, Barratt-Boyes and Lowe, 1961). It is also known as infantile hypercalcaemia, because children have abnormalities in the metabolism of calcium and calcitonin. Other clinical features include a failure to thrive in the first year of life. The 'elfin' face includes a star-like pattern on the iris, the growth of the eyebrow hair towards the nose which is upturned at the end, thick lips and an open-mouth posture. A mixed pattern of development has been found in the groups of individuals studied and there is some suggestion that their general cognitive abilities (usually in the IQ range 45–55) are mismatched with their language skills which appear, on the surface at least, to be rather better (Bellugi et al., 1988).

Worster-Drought Syndrome

This is also called congenital suprabulbar paresis, and was described by Worster-Drought in 1956. It is a severe, non-progressive motor speech impairment. As the name implies the lesion is situated above the brain stem, pons and medulla, in the motor tract between the motor cortex to the nuclei of the tenth and twelfth cranial nerves. The syndrome may be familial. A history of poor sucking and swallowing is usual. The usual neurological manifestation is a weakness and spasticity of the lips (orbicularis oris muscle), tongue, soft palate and, when more severe, of the pharyngeal and laryngeal muscles. The combination of muscles affected and the severity may vary. There is usually a brisk jaw jerk. At best speech is hypernasal, slurred and indistinct, but in the more severe cases there may be little or no movement of the articulators. In this form there is usually a difficulty in swallowing and little or no phonation. The child commonly has difficulty controlling saliva and drools persistently. In its mildest form, it may be restricted to a weakness of the soft palate. An acquired form of suprabulbar paresis is rarer but may be subsequent to encephalitis or other acquired cerebral lesions.

Appendix II
Scripts for Story
Telling

These are the complete texts of the Dog Story and the Farmer Story as told to the children for the Story Telling tasks. The method is that recommended by Mandler and Johnson (1977). Unfortunately norms are not yet available. However, the technique can be used successfully with most children of 6 years and over to elicit a short expressive language sample. The episode numbers refer to the major components of each story. A ratio of episode numbers (e.g. 8 out of 11) could be used to give an indication of how much of the story was accurately recalled. The stories should be told at an even pace, without any undue emphasis, but in as natural a manner as possible. The child should then be asked to retell the story and can be cued if necessary. It is recommmended that the child's response be tape recorded for later transcription and any cues given should be marked. These stories can form a useful point of departure for subsequent conversation, particularly if the child is reluctant to converse spontaneously.

Complete Dog Story

Episode number

1	There was a dog who had a piece of meat
2	and he was carrying it home in his mouth.
3	On the way home he had to cross a bridge across a stream.
4	As he crossed he looked down
5	and saw his reflection in the water.
6	He thought it was another dog with another piece of meat
7	and he wanted to have that piece as well.
8	So he tried to bite the reflection
9	but as he opened his mouth his piece of meat fell out,
10	dropped into the water,
11	and was never seen again.

Complete Farmer Story

Episode number

1	Once there was an old farmer
2	who owned a very stubborn donkey.
3	One evening, the farmer wanted to put his donkey into the barn.
4	First he pushed him,
5	but the donkey would not move.
6	Then he pulled him,
7	but the donkey still would not move.
8	Next the farmer thought he could frighten the donkey into the barn.
9	So he asked the dog to bark at the donkey,
10	but the lazy dog refused.
11	Then the farmer thought that the cat could get the dog to bark.
12	So he asked the cat to scratch the dog.
13	The cooperative cat scratched the dog.
14	The dog immediately began to bark.
15	The barking so frightened the donkey
16	that he jumped into the barn.

References

ACARDI, J and CHEVRIE, J.J. (1986). Children with epilepsy. In: Gordon, N. and McKinley, I. (Eds) *Neurologically Handicapped Children: Treatment and Management*. Oxford: Blackwell.

ADAMS, C. and BISHOP, D.V.M. (1989). Conversational characteristics of children with semantic–pragmatic disorder I: Exchange structure, turn taking, repairs and cohesion. *British Journal of Disorders of Communication* 24, 211–213.

ASPERGER, M. (1944). Die 'Autistischen Psychopathen' im Kindesalter. *Archiv für Psychiatrie und Nervenkrankenteiten* 117, 76–136.

AVRAHAMI, E., HAREL, S., JURGENSON, U. and COHN, D.F. (1985). Computed tomographic demonstration of brain changes in Incontinentia Pigmenti. *American Journal of Disorders in Childhood*. 139, 372–374.

BARNES, D. (1969). Language in the secondary classroom. In: Barnes, D., Britton, J and Rossen, H. (Eds), *Language, the Learner and the School*, pp. 9–78. Harmondsworth: Penguin Education.

BARNES, D., BRITTON, J and ROSSEN, H. (Eds) (1969). *Language, the Learner and the School*. Harmondsworth: Penguin Education.

BATES, E., BENIGNI, L, BRETHERTON, I., CAMAIONI, L and VOLTERRA, V. (1979). *The Emergence of Symbols: Communication and cognition in infancy*. New York: Academic Press.

BAX, M.C.O. (1964). Terminology and classification of cerebral palsy. *Developmental Medicine and Child Neurology* 6, 296–297.

BELLUGI, U., MARKS, S., BIHRLE, A. and SABO, H. (1988). Dissociation between language and cognitive function in Williams Syndrome. In: Bishop, D. and Mogford, K. (Eds), *Language Development in Exceptional Circumstances*. Edinburgh: Churchill Livingstone.

BISHOP, D.V.M. (1979). Comprehension in developmental language disorders. *Developmental Medicine and Child Neurology* 21, 225–238.

BISHOP, D.V.M. (1982). Comprehension of spoken, written and signed sentences in childhood language disorders. *Journal of Child Psychology and Psychiatry*, 23(1), 1–20.

BISHOP, D.V.M. (1983). *The Test for Reception of Grammar*. Published by the author at the University of Manchester, Oxford Road, Manchester M13 9PL.

BISHOP, D.V.M. (1984). Automated LARSP: computer assisted grammatical analysis. *British Journal of Disorders of Communication* 19, 78–87.

BISHOP, D.V.M. (1985). Age of onset and outcome in 'Acquired Aphasia with Convulsive

224

Disorder' (Landau–Kleffner Syndrome). *Developmental Medicine and Child Neurology* 27, 705–712.

BISHOP, D.V.M. (1987). The causes of specific developmental language disorder. *Journal of Child Psychology and Psychiatry* 28, 1–8.

BISHOP, D.V.M. (1987). The concept of comprehension in language disorder. *Proceedings of the First International Symposium of Specific Speech and Language Disorders in Childhood.* London: AFASIC.

BISHOP, D.V.M. (1988). Language development after focal brain injury. In Bishop, D. and Mogford, K. (Eds), *Language Development in Exceptional Circumstances.* Edinburgh: Churchill Livingstone.

BISHOP, D.V.M. (1989). Autism, Asperger's syndrome and semantic–prgamatic disorder: Where are the boundaries? *British Journal of Disorders of Communication* 24, 107–122.

BISHOP, D.V.M. and ADAMS, C. (1989). Conversational characteristics of children with semantic–pragmatic disorders II: What features lead to a judgement of inappropriacy? *British Journal of Disorders of Communication* 24, 241–264.

BISHOP, .D.V.M and EDMUNDSON, A. (1987). Specific language impairment as a maturational lag; evidence from longitudinal data on language and motor development. *Developmental Medicine and Child Neurology* 29, 442–459.

BISHOP, D.V.M and MOGFORD, K. (Eds) (1988). *Language Development in Exceptional Circumstances.* Edinburgh: Churchill Livingstone.

BISHOP, D.V.M and ROSENBLOOM, L. (1987). Classification of childhood language disorders. In Yule, W. and Rutter, M. (Eds), *Language Development and Disorders.* Oxford: McKeith Press (Blackwell).

BLOOM, L. and LAHEY, M. (1978). *Language Development and Language Disorders.* New York: John Wiley and Sons.

BOEHM, A. (1971). *The Boehm Test of Basic Concepts.* London: Psychological Corporation & Harcourt, Brace, Jovanovich.

BOEHM, A. (1986). *The Boehm Test of Basic Concepts* (revised). London: Psychological Corporation & Harcourt, Brace, Jovanovich.

BOWERMAN, M. (1982). Process of lexical and syntactic development in language acquisition. In: *Language Acquisition, the State of the Art.* Cambridge: Cambridge University Press.

BRACKEN, B. (1984). *Bracken Basic Concepts Scale.* London: Psychological Corporation, Harcourt, Brace & Jovanovich.

BROCA, P. (1863). Localisation des fonctions cerebrales: siège du langage articule. *Bulletin de la Société d'Anthropologie* 4, 200–204.

BUDDEN, S., MEEK, M. and HENIGAN, C. (1990). Communication and oral-motor function in Rett's Syndrome. *Developmental Medicine and Child Neurology* 32, 51–55.

BZOCH, K.R. and LEAGUE, R. (1970). *The Receptive and Expressive Emergent Language Scale.* Baltimore: University Park Press.

CARROW, E. (1974). *Carrow Elicited Language Inventory.* Texas: Learning Concepts.

CHADWICK, O., RUTTER, M., THOMPSON, J. and SCHAFFER, D. (1981). Intellectual performance and reading skills after localised head injury in childhood. *Journal of Child Psychology and Psychiatry* 22, 117–139.

CHIAT, S. and HIRSON, A. (1987). From conceptual intention to utterance: a study of impaired language output in a child with developmental dysphasia. *British Journal of Disorders of Communication* 22, 37–64.

CLEZY, G. (1978). The modification of the mother–child interchange. *British Journal of Disorders of Communication* 113, 93–106.

COLLIGNON, R., HECAEN, H. and ANGELERGUES, G. (1968). A propos de 12 cas d'aphasie acquise de l'enfant. *Acta Neurologica et Psychiatrica Belgica* **68**, 245–277.

COMPTON, A.J. (1976). Generative studies of children's phonological disorders: clinical ramifications. In: Morehead, D.M. and Morehead, A.E. (Eds), *Normal and Deficient Child Language*. Baltimore: University Park Press.

COOK, J. and WILLIAMS, D. (1985). *Working with Children's Language*. Oxon: Winslow Press.

COOMBES, K. (1987). Speech therapy. In: Yule, W. and Rutter, M. (Eds), *Language Development and Disorders*. Oxford: McKeith Press (Blackwell).

COOPER, J.A. and FERRY, P.C. (1978). Acquired auditory verbal agnosia and seizures in childhood. *Journal of Speech and Hearing Disorders* **43**, 176–184.

COOPER, J.A. and FLOWERS, C.R. (1987). Children with a history of acquired aphasia: residual language and academic impairments. *Journal of Speech and Hearing Disorders* **52**, 251–262.

COOPER, J., MOODLEY, M. and REYNELL, J. (1978). *Helping Language Development*. London: Edward Arnold.

CORBETT, J. (1985). Epilepsy as part of a handicapping condition. In: Ross, E. and Reynolds, E. (Eds), *Paediatric Perspectives on Epilepsy*. Chichester: J. Wiley and Sons.

CRYSTAL, D. (1982a). *Profiling Language Disability* London: Edward Arnold.

CRYSTAL, D. (1982b). Time, terms and teeth – Eslie Fogarty Lecture. *British Journal of Disorders of Communication* **17**, 3–19.

CRYSTAL, D., FLETCHER, P. and GARMAN, M. (1976). *The Grammatical Analysis of Language Disability*. London: Edward Arnold.

DALTON, C. (1989). *An expert system for diagnosis*. Unpublished MSc dissertation, Birbeck College, University of London.

DEAN, E and HOWELL, J. (1986). Developing linguistic awareness: a theoretically based approach to phonological disorders. *British Journal of Disorders of Communication* **21**, 223–238.

DEONNA, T., BEAUMANIOR, A., GAILLARD, F. and ASSAL, G. (1977). Acquired aphasia in childhood with seizure disorder; a heteogeneous syndrome. *Neuropaediatrie* **8**(3), 263–273.

DEWART, H. and SUMMERS, S. (1988). *The Pragmatic Profile of Early Communication Skills*. Windsor: NFER.

DORE, J. (1975). Holophrases, speech acts and language universals. *Journal of Child Language* **2**, 21–40.

DOWLING, M. (1980). *Early Projects*. Harlow: Longman Early Childhood Education.

DOWN, J.L.H. (1866). Observations on an ethnic classification of idiots. *London Hospital Reports* 259.

DUGAS, M., GRENET, P., MASSON, M., MIALET, J.P. and JAQUET, G. (1976). Aphasie de l'enfant avec epilepsie; evolution regressive sous traitement antiepileptique. *Revue Neurologique (Paris)* **132**(7), 489–493.

DULAC, O., BILLARD, C. and ARTHUIS, M. (1983). Aspects electro-cliniques et evolutivs de l'epilepsie dans le syndrome aphasie-epilepsie. *Archives Françaises Pediatrie (Paris)* **40**, 299–308.

EASTWOOD, J. (1986). Qualitative research: An additional research methodology for speech pathology? *British Journal of Disorders of Communication* **23**, 171–184.

ENDERBY, P. (1983). *The Frenchay Dysarthria Test*. Windsor: NFER.

EWING-COBBS, L., FLETCHER, J.M., LANDRY, S.H. and LEVIN, H.S. (1985). Language disorders after paediatric head injury. In: *Speech and Language Evaluation in Neurology: Childhood Disorders*. New York: Grune & Stratton.

FAWCUS, M., ROBINSON, M., WILLIAMS, J. and WILLIAMS, R. (1983). *Working with Dysphasics*. Oxon: Winslow Press.

FOX, J., ALVEY, P. and MYERS, C. (1983). Decision technology and man-machine interaction. *Proceedings of Expert Systems Conference*, Cambridge.

FRENCH, A. (1989). Can children with semantic–pragmatic disorders learn a task if it is structured into small steps, and are they able to generalise this? Unpublished BSc project. Department of Clinical Communication Studies, City University, London.

FUNDUDIS, T., KOLVIN, I. and GARSIDE, R.F. (1979). *Speech Retarded and Deaf Children: Their Psychological Development*. London: Academic Press.

GADDES, W.H. and CROCKETT, D.J. (1975). The Spreen–Benton aphasia tests; normative data as a measure of language development. *Brain and Language 2*, 257–280.

GALLAGHER, T.M. and PRUTTING, C. (1983). *Pragmatic Assessment and Intervention Issues in Language*. San Diego: College Hill Press.

GARVEY, C. (1982). *Play*. New York: Fontana Publications.

GERARD, K. (1986). *The Checklist of Communicative Competence*. Available from the author at 3 Perry mansions, 113 Catford Hill, London SE6.

GERMAN, D.J. (1985). The use of specific semantic word categories in the diagnosis of dysnomic learning-disabled children. *British Journal of Disorders of Communication 20*, 143–154.

GERMAN, D.J. (1986). *National College of Education Test of Word Finding (TWF)*. Allen, TX: DLM Teaching Resources.

GERMAN, D.J. (1989). A diagnostic model and a test to assess word-finding skills in children. *British Journal of Disorders of Communication 24*, 21–39.

GOODGLASS, H. and KAPLAN, E. (1972). *The Assessment of Aphasia and Related Disorders*. Philadelphia: Lea and Febiger.

GOODMAN, R. (1987). The developmental neurobiology of language. In: Yule, W. and Rutter, M. (Eds), *Language Development and Disorders*. Oxford: Mackeith Press (Blackwell).

GORDON, N. and McKINLAY, I. (1980). *Helping Clumsy Children*. Edinburgh: Churchill Livingstone.

GRIFFITHS, P. (1969). A follow up of children with disorders of speech. *British Journal of Disorders of Communication 4*, 46–56.

GRIFFITHS, R. (1954). *The Abilities of Babies*. Windsor: NFER.

GRIFFITHS, R. (1970). *The Abilities of Young Children*. Windsor: NFER.

GUTTMAN, E. (1942). Aphasia in children. *Brain 65*, 205–219.

HARRIS, D.B. (1963). *Children's drawings as measures of intellectual maturity; a revision and extension of the Goodenough Draw a Man Test*. New York: Harcourt, Brace and World.

HAYNES, C. (1982). *Vocabulary acquisition problems in language disordered children*. Unpublished MSc Thesis, City University, London.

HAYNES, C. (1986). Semantic and Pragmatic Colloquim. Available from the author at Dawn House School, Nottingham.

HECAEN, H. (1976). Acquired aphasia in children and the ontogenesis of hemispheric specialization. *Brain and Language 3*, 114–134.

HOPKINS-ACOS, P and BUNKER, K. (1979). A child with Noonan Syndrome. *Journal of Speech and Hearing Disorders 44*, 494–503.

HOWARD, D., PATTERSON, K.E., FRANKLIN, S., ORCHARD-LISLE, V.M. and MORTON, J. (1985). Treatment of word retrevial deficits in aphasia; a comparison of two therapy methods. *Brain 108*, 817–829.

HUTT, E. (1986). *Teaching Language Disordered Children: A structured curriculum*.

London: Edward Arnold.

JARVIS, J. (1989). Taking a Metaphon approach to phonological development: a case study. *Child Language Teaching and Therapy* **5**, 16–32.

JEFFREE, D., McKONKY, R. and HEWSON, S. (1977). *Let me Play.* London: Human Horizons Series, Souvenir Press.

JOHNSTON, J. and RAMSTAD, V. (1983). Cognitive development in pre-adolescent language impaired children. *British Journal of Disorders of Communication,* **18**, 49–55.

JONES, S. (1987). Paget Gorman Signed Speech. *Proceedings of the First International Symposium; Specific Speech and Language Disorders.* London: AFASIC.

JORDAN, F.M., OZANNE, A.E. and MURDOCH, B.E. (1988). Long-term speech and language disorder subsequent to closed head injury in children. *Brain Injury* **2**, 179–185.

KANNER, L. (1943). Autistic disturbance of affective contact. *Nervous Child* **2**, 217–250.

KAZDIN, A.E. (1982). *Single Case Research Designs.* Oxford: Oxford University Press.

KELLETT, B. and WARD, S. (1980). Language disordered or deaf? *British Journal of Disorders of Communication* **15**, 31–39.

KIRK, A.S., McCARTHY, J.J. and KIRK, W.D. (1968). *The Illinois Test of Psycholinguistic Abilities.* University of Illinois.

KIRK, S.A. and KIRK, W. (1971). *GOAL: A remediation programme for children with psycholinguistic abilities.* Windsor: NFER.

KLINEFELTER, H.F., REIFENSTEIN, E.C. and ALBRIGHT, F. (1942). Syndrome characterised by gynecomastia, aspermatogenesis without aleydigism and increased secretion of follicle-stimulating hormone (gynecomastia). *Journal of Clinical Endrocrinology and Metabolism* **2**, 615.

KNOWLES, W. and MASIDLOVER, M. (1982). *The Derbyshire Language Scheme.* Education Office, Grosvenor road, Ripley, Derbyshire.

KRATOCHWILL, T.R. (1978). *Single Subject Research.* London: Academic Press.

LANDAU, W.M. and KLEFFNER, F. (1957). Syndrome of acquired aphasia with convulsive disorder in children. *Neurology* **7**, 523–530.

LEA, J. (1970). The colour pattern scheme: a method of remedial language teaching. Moor House School, Oxted, Surrey.

LEA, J. (1980). Rhythmic ability and language ability. In: Jones, F.M. (Ed), *Language Disability in Children.* Lancaster: MTP Press.

LEES, J.A. (1989). *A linguistic investigation of acquired childhood aphasia.* Unpublished MPhil thesis, City University, London.

LEITER, R. (1969). *Leiter International Performance Scale.* Chicago: Stoelting Co.

LEONARD, L.B. (1979). Language impairment in children. *Merrill Palmer Quarterly* **25** (3), 205–230.

LEVIN, H.S., MADDISON, C.F., BAILEY, C.B., MEYERS, C.A., EISENBERG, H.M. and GUINTO, F.C. (1983). Mutism after closed head injury. *Archives of Neurology* **40**, 601–606.

LOCKE, A. (1980). *Living Language.* Windsor: NFER.

LOWE, M. and COSTELLO, A. (1976). *The Symbolic Play Test.* Windsor: NFER.

LUBS, H.A. (1983). X-linked mental retardation and the marker X. In: Emery, E. and Rimoin, D. (Eds), *Principles and Practice of Medical Genetics.* Edinburgh: Churchill Livingstone.

McDADE, H.L. (1981). A parent–child interaction model for assessing and remediating language disability. *British Journal of Disorders of Communication* **16**, 175–183.

McKENNA, P. and WARRINGTON, E. (1983). *The Graded Naming Test.* Windsor: NFER.

McMILLEN, M.E., MULE, L.N. and LEES, J.A. (1987). Acquired Neurological Insult in children; current management issues – USA/UK. Presented at the Eighth Annual Traumatic Head Injury programme, Braintree, Massachusetts.

McTEAR, M.F. (1985). *Children's Conversation*. Oxford: Blackwell.

McTEAR, M.F. (1985). Pragmatic disorders: a question of direction. *British Journal of Disorders of Communication* **20**, 119–127.

MANDLER, J.M. and JOHNSON, N.S. (1977). Remembrance of things parsed: Story structure and recall. *Cognitive Psychology* **8**, 111–151.

MARSHALL, J. (1986). The description and interpretation of aphasic language disorder. *Neuropsychologia* **24**, 5–24.

MARTIN, J.A.M. (1984). Syndrome delineation in communication disorders. In: Herson, L.A. and Berger, M. (Eds), *Language and Language Disorders in Childhood*. Oxford: Pergamon Press.

MARTLEW, M. (1987). Prelinguistic communication. In: Yule, W. and Rutter, M. (Eds), *Language Development and Disorders*. Oxford: McKeith Press (Blackwell).

MULLER, D.J. (1984). What does a language score really mean? *Journal of Child Language Teaching and Therapy* **1**, 38–45.

MULLER, D.J., MUNRO, X. and CODE, C. (1981). *Language Assessment for Remediation*. London: Croom-Helm.

NEWCOMER, P., HARE, B., HAMMILL, D. and McGETTIGAN, J. (1973). *Construct Validity of ITPA*. Tuscon: Arizona University Press.

NEWTON, A. and THOMPSON, M. (1976). *The Aston Index*. Wisbech: Learning Development Aids.

NOONAN, J.A. and EHMKE, D.A. (1963). Associated noncardiac malformations in children with congenital heart disease. *Journal of Pediatrics* **63**, 468–470.

PAGET, R., GORMAN, P. and PAGET, G. (1976). *The Paget Gorman Sign System*. Association for Experiment in Deaf Education, London.

PENFIELD, W. and RASMUSSEN, T. (1950). *The Cerebral Cortex of Man*. London: Macmillan.

POCKLINGTON, S. and HEGARTY, K. (1981). *Educating Pupils with Special Needs in the Ordinary School*. Windsor: NFER.

POCKLINGTON, S. and HEGARTY, K. (1982). *The Development of a Language Unit: Rose Hill, Oxford*. Windsor: NFER.

POCKLINGTON, S. and HEGARTY, K. (1982). *Integration in Action*. Windsor: NFER.

PORCH, B. (1972). *The Porch Index of Communicative Ability in Children*. Palo Alto: Consulting Psychologists Press.

PRING, T. (1987). On choosing a methodology to assess the efecctiveness of therapeutic intervention: a reply to FitzGibbon. *British Journal of Disorders of Communication* **22**, 163–166.

RAPIN, I. and ALLEN, D.A. (1987). Developmental dysphasia and autism in preschool children: Characteristics and subtypes. *Proceedings of the First International Symposium on Speech and Language Disorders in Children*. London: AFASIC.

RENFEW, C. (1972a). *The Action Picture Test*. Published by the author at North Place, Old Headington, Oxford.

RENFEW, C. (1972b). *The Bus Story Test*. Published by the author at North Place, Old Headington, Oxford.

RENFEW, C. (1972c). *The Word Finding Vocabulary Test*. Published by the author at North Place, Old Headington, Oxford.

RETT, A. (1966). *Über ein zerebral-atrophisches Syndrom bei Hyperammonamie*. Wein: Bruder Hollinek.

REYNELL, J. (1977). *The Reynell Developmental Language Scales*. Windsor: NFER.

REYNELL, J. (1980). *Language Development and Assessment*. Lancaster: MTP Press.

REYNELL, J. (1985). *The Reynell Developmental Language Scales – Revised*. Windsor: NFER.

RIPLEY, K. and LEA, J. (1984). Moor House School: a follow up study of receptive aphasic ex-pupils. Moor House School, Oxted, Surrey.

ROBINSON, R.J. (1987). The causes of language disorder: introduction and overview. *Proceedings of the First International Symposium of Specific Speech and Language Disorders in Children*, Reading, England. London: AFASIC.

RONDAL, J.A. (1988). Down's syndrome. In: Bishop, D. and Mogford, K. (Eds), *Language Development in Exceptional Circumstances*. Edinburgh: Churchill Livingstone.

ROUX, J. and SCHNEIDER, C. (1988). Refer to Specific Interest Group (Language Units) ILEA. John Ruskin Language Unit, John Ruskin Street, London SE5.

RUTTER, M. (1978a). Diagnosis and definition. In: Rutter, M. and Schopler, E. (Eds), *Autism: A Reappraisal of concepts and treatment*. New York: Plenum Press.

RUTTER, M. (1978b). Language disorder and infantile autism. In: Rutter, M. and Schopler, E. (Eds), *Autism: A reappraisal of concepts and treatment*. New York: Plenum Press.

SCHIEFELBUSCH, R.L. and PIKAR, J. (1986). *Language Competence: Assessment and Intervention*. London: Taylor & Francis.

SEMEL, E. and WIIG, E. (1987). *Clinical Evaluation of Language Functions*. London: Psychological Corporation, Harcourt Brace Jovanovich.

SHERIDAN, M. (1973). *Children's Developmental Progress from Birth to Five Years: the Stycar sequences*. Windsor: NFER.

SHERIDAN, M. (1977). *Spontaneous Play in Early Childhood, from Birth to Six Years*. Windsor: NFER.

SILVA, P.A., McGEE, R.O. and WILLIAMS, S.M. (1983). Developmental language delay from three to seven years and its significance for low intelligence and reading difficulties at age seven. *Developmental Medicine and Child Neurology* 25, 783–793.

SMITH, P.A. and MARX, R.W. (1971). The factor structure of the revised addition of ITPA. *Psychology in Schools* 8, 349–356.

SPREEN, O. and BENTON, A.L. (1969). *Neurosensory Center Comprehensive Examination for Aphasia*. Neuropsychology Laboratory, University of Victoria, Victoria.

STEVENSON, J. (1984). Predictive value of speech and language screening. *Developmental Medicine and Child Neurology* 26, 528–538.

STEVENSON, J. and RICHMAN, N. (1976). The prevalence of language delay in a population of three year old children and its association with general retardation. *Developmental Medicine and Child Neurology* 18, 431–441.

STEVENSON, P., BAX, M. and STEVENSON, J. (1982). The evaluation of home based speech therapy for language delayed preschool children in an inner city area. *British Journal of Disorders of Communication* 17, 141–148.

TALLAL, P., STARK, R.E. and MELLITIS, E.D. (1985). The relationship between auditory temporal analysis and receptive language development; evidence from studies of developmental language disorder. *Neuropsychologia* 23, 527–533.

THOMSON, M. (1984). *Developmental Dyslexia*. London: Edward Arnold.

TURNER, M. and VINCENT, C. (1987). Are speech and language units effective? *Educational Psychology in Practice* (April), 36–41.

UDWIN, O. and YULE, W. (1983). Imaginative play in language disordered children. *British Journal of Disorders of Communication* 18, 197–205.

URWIN, S., COOK, J. and KELLY, K. (1988). Pre-school language intervention; a follow up study. *Child Care Health and Development* 14, 127–146.

VAN DER SANDT-KOENDERMAN, W.M.E., SMIT, I.A.C., VAN DONGEN, H.R. and VAN HEST, J.B.C. (1984). A case of acquired aphasia with convulsive disorder: some linguistic aspects of recovery and breakdown. *Brain and Language* 21, 174–183.

VAN DONGEN, H.R., LOONEN, McB. and VAN DONGEN, K.J. (1985). Anatomical basis for acquired fluent aphasia in children. *Annals of Neurology* **17**(3), 306–309.

VAN HOUT, A., EVRARD, P. and LYON, G. (1985). On the positive semiology of acquired aphasia in children. *Developmental Medicine and Child Neurology* **27**, 231–241.

WALKER, M. (1980). *The Revised Makaton Vocabulary*. Published by the author, St George's Hospital, London.

WARD, S. (1984). Detecting abnormal behaviours in infancy: the relation between such behaviours and linguistic development. *British Journal of Disorders of Communication* **19**, 237–251.

WARD, S. and KELLET, B. (1982). Language disorder resolved? *British Journal of Disorders of Communication* **17**, 33–52.

WECHSLER, D. (1974). *The Wechsler Intelligence Scale for Children – Revised (WISC-R)*. New York: The Psychological Corporation.

WHURR, R. and EVANS, S. (1986). *The Children's Aphasia Screening Test*. Published by the authors at the National Hospital for Nervous Diseases, London.

WIIG, E.H. (1987). Strategic language use in adolescents with learning disabilities: Assessment and education. In: *Proceedings of First International Symposium, Specific Speech and Language Disorders in Children*. London: AFASIC.

WIIG, E.H. and SECORD, W. (1986). Diagnostic validity of Test of Language competence for LLD adolescents. Paper presented at the Annual Convention of ASHA, Detroit.

WILLIAMS, J.C.P., BARRATT-BOYES, B.G. and LOWE, J.B. (1961). Supravalvular aortic stenosis. *Circulation* **24**, 1311–1318.

WILSON, M. and DYSON, A. (1982). Noonan Syndrome: Speech and language characteristics. *Journal of Communication Disorders* **15**, 347–352.

WING, L. (1981). Language, social and cognitive impairments in autism and severe mental retardation. *Journal of Autism and Developmental Disorders* **11**, 31–44.

WORSTER-DROUGHT, C. (1956). Congenital suprabulbar paresis. *Journal of Laryngology and Otology* **70**, 453–463.

Index